Advance Praise

"*Why Can't I Stick to my Diet?* It's a universal question. Yo-yo dieting has almost been elevated to the status of the law of gravity – a foregone conclusion. Erin has finally shattered these outdated ideas and replaced them with ones that work. She's not an ivory-tower academic spouting theories she's never lived. Her story in Chapter One, *My Life, My Weight, and What I Ate*, will make you alternately laugh and cry. The story is one I've heard thousands of times- and seen myself in. I guarantee you will see yourself in the pages of this book. More importantly, she shares her mental process and path as she begins to put together the pieces that eventually change her life. Her brutal self-honesty, self-depreciating humor, and the fact that she is willing to share it all openly makes reading her story a joy.

"If I could craft a perfect counselor for people with sugar and weight issues it would be Erin. Her background in holistic nutrition coaching is perfect for motivating and delivering information about food and diet in a succinct and relatable way. You will put this book down with a complete understanding of how what you put in your mouth is related to how you feel, and what to do to change this behavior. This book and your association with Erin and her community will lead you to a deeper understanding of WHY you've not had success in the past and just exactly how you can change all that starting right now."

MICHAEL COLLINS
Founder
SugarAddiction.com
Author of *The Last Resort Sugar Detox*

"*Why Can't I Stick to my Diet* is the most helpful book that I have read about food in a long time. As someone who has always struggled with weight and wellness, I found such encouragement in Erin's authenticity and transparency about her own struggles. She educates with compassion but pulls no punches. If you've ever struggled with food like I have, the concrete, no bull approach Erin provides is priceless.

"She takes the complicated science of nutrition (which I find baffling even though I am a trained scientist myself) and explains it in a practical and useful way. I need to know the "why" for the changes that I am asked to make. Erin shows us the why and but goes further, asking us to develop our own solid reasons for ditching sugar. Then she uses her own story to demonstrate the payoffs. I encourage anyone who has ever struggled to stick with healthy eating to read this book. If your health is like mine when I first read it, you have nothing to lose and possibly so much to gain."

DR. RACHEL MORRIS
PhD Biological Sciences
Michigan State University

"Erin brings her experience as a Holistic Health Coach and a Food Addiction Counselor to give us an honest, how-to, practical guide to eliminating sugar, flour, and sweeteners from our diets. If you go from diet to diet and just can't beat your cravings, this is the book for you."

DR. MICHAEL GELB DDS, MD
New York, New York
Author of *Gasp!: Airway Health -*
The Hidden Path To Wellness

Why Can't I Stick to My Diet?

Why Can't I Stick To My DIET?

Feel Better, Look Good and Never Ask That Question Again

Erin Boardman Wathen

NEW YORK

LONDON • NASHVILLE • MELBOURNE • VANCOUVER

Why Can't I Stick to My Diet?
Feel Better, Look Good and Never Ask That Question Again

© 2019 Erin Boardman Wathen

Published in New York, New York, by Morgan James Publishing in partnership with Difference Press. Morgan James is a trademark of Morgan James, LLC. www.MorganJamesPublishing.com

The Morgan James Speakers Group can bring authors to your live event. For more information or to book an event visit The Morgan James Speakers Group at www.TheMorganJamesSpeakersGroup.com.

ISBN 9781683509998 paperback
ISBN 9781642790009 eBook
Library of Congress Control Number: 2018935524

Cover Design by:
Megan Dillon
megan@creativeninjadesigns.com

Interior Design by:
Chris Treccani
www.3dogcreative.net

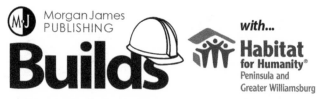

In an effort to support local communities, raise awareness and funds, Morgan James Publishing donates a percentage of all book sales for the life of each book to Habitat for Humanity Peninsula and Greater Williamsburg.

Get involved today! Visit
www.MorganJamesBuilds.com

For my husband, who has always believed in me.

For my kids, to whom I have been promising a trip to Disney World

when I finally finish this book.

Foreword
by JJ Virgin

WHY CAN'T I STICK TO MY DIET? It is a question many of us have asked but what is the real answer? Willpower, finding the right diet, doctor or spending more money on magic potions?

Erin Boardman Wathen answers this age old question with a sensible approach to food and a logical way of looking at life. Erin answers this question without shame or finger pointing. It is as if Erin has cracked the code and is sharing it with a close girlfriend over a cup of tea after school drop off.

So many women struggle with their weight and Erin gets to the root cause of why we gained it in the first place. Her personal experience along with her education makes her a great guide into why we regain weight and how to make sure it doesn't happen in the future. Her loving, no nonsense approach combined with self deprecating humor and pop culture references will keep you motivated and interested until the last page.

Sugar addiction, is often misunderstood and it is a problem for so many of us. Erin is able to explain the science in a way that makes sense and is relatable. You will understand the reason why Sugar hijacks your brain, as Erin calls it, and know it is not your body demanding more

Sugar once you have indulged, it is the Sugar! She is able to lovingly tell us why just because a food looks healthy, it might not be or that the beloved treats you grew up with might not be an option any longer.

There are always those women in our lives, who seem to effortlessly maintain their weight. Maybe we know them as another parent from our kids lacrosse team, or we went to college with them, or they are a friend from work. These women workout because they enjoy it, and they know how important it is for stress relief and to connect with their body, not because they want to undo a caloric indulgence. They never talk about the latest fat diet, or an extreme way they plan on losing weight before the next bathing suit situation. They are simply living, and maintain a healthy weight, where their body wants to be, without any tricks or schemes. Can you imagine how that must feel? It is all possible. We all want to get to our real, natural weight and get on with life.

Congratulations on picking up Erin's book and starting your journey into a life without stressing about whether or not your jeans will fit on Friday, or if you will ever be able to stick to your diet.

JJ VIRGIN, CNS, CHFS
Celebrity Nutrition & Fitness Expert
4xNYT Bestselling Author including
The Virgin Diet & The Sugar Impact Diet

Table of Contents

Introduction

Food is our common ground, a universal experience.

– James Beard

I WAKE UP, and for a good 30 seconds my mind is clear and I do not immediately start to replay what I ate the night before. I am simply thinking of what my day will bring. Then, I remember what I did in the kitchen … the ice cream, the cookies, the leftover cupcakes from the kids' party. CRAAAAAP, did I really eat all of that? I touch my stomach, and wow, am I bloated! I lick my teeth and they still taste sweet. I must have been so out of it I didn't brush my teeth before I went to bed. Wait, I think I have a little bit of cake in the back of my mouth. YUCK.

Thankfully, my husband snores, so I had slept in the guest room last night as a preventative measure. Let's be honest here, the sleeping arrangement gave me privacy to do my secret food thing at night. I go down to our bedroom and notice how dry my mouth is. I slowly open the door. My husband is still sleeping, and the clock next to him shows there's still nine minutes before the alarm will go off. I never sleep well when I eat at night.

I go into the bathroom and get a look at myself. My face is pretty swollen and I contemplate weighing myself to see if any of the damage "took" or not. I figure I still can keep eating since I haven't brushed my teeth. But then I get on the scale. YIKES. I step off the scale and take off all of my clothes, silently praying my husband or daughter doesn't barge into the bathroom and question why I am totally naked and getting on and off the scale like it is a Magic 8 Ball that will eventually give me the right answer. I guess I am up a good 3.5 pounds since last week. I must be retaining water or something. It can't be *real* weight, right? I look at myself in the mirror. I am super puffy in the middle. It is not a cute look. I throw on my pajamas and admit defeat by brushing my teeth, going to get my youngest out of his crib, and heading for the stairs. I'm grateful the coffee pot knows what time it is.

What happened that got me into the food? I wish I could remember. I put my two-year-old down in front of *Sesame Street*, then head into the kitchen to grab the biggest coffee mug I can find in the cabinet. It must be size of my head. I pour in a bunch of fat-free milk and then as many packets of artificial sweetener as I can find. The white stuff sprays all over the place and I stir as quickly as I can. I down the entire mug by the time my five-year-old pads down the stairs in her nightgown. She demands French toast, which is the last thing I want to make. My food hangover is in full effect.

As I cook, I start planning how little I will eat today to make up for all the sugar I ate last night. I will do a double spin class when my daughter is at preschool and the sitter has come over to watch my son. All I will eat is protein and water. I will be back to normal in time for the weekend, since today is only Tuesday. I don't want to have to call in Fat for our dinner plans with our friends. I did that a few months ago and it was so embarrassing, which only led me to eat more sugar. I am too old for this crap.

Time to flip the stupid French toast. The kids are bickering over something. My husband comes downstairs asking about the dry cleaning and why the dog is barking. Where is my stinking coffee? I add more skim milk and sweetener. My head has started to hurt, so I toss some Advil down with the coffee.

Time to get moving for school. I need to leave in 20 minutes or so to drop off my daughter, then go to spin to do a double, go to the grocery store to get healthy food, then I have a meeting or something later. I really can't think today, who was I supposed to call? Damn, I wish I'd written it down. I hope it will come to me.

I start to clear the dishes, and as I am about to toss the leftover French toast into the trash, I furtively eat the cold slices. I can hear my husband is in the shower. The sitter will be here in ten minutes, and my toddler is, for the moment, busy with his iPad and facing the other direction. I eat over the trash as quickly as I can. WAIT! I wasn't going to eat anything bad today, much less maple syrup and bread cooked in butter! What is wrong with me? Seriously, when will I ever learn??

The sitter finally shows, and my husband asks me to do five different things on his way out the door. Like I do not have anything better to do! Who was I supposed to call again? My daughter and I head out to the car, and I grab more coffee in a travel mug. Caffeine will help me when I work out! My exercise clothes feel super tight across my waist, and I feel disgusting as I drive to school. Tons of traffic and really awful mommy drivers. I head to the gym and my head is killing me. I can't tell if it is from too much coffee or last night or if I am getting sick. I walk into spin and try to avoid eye contact with my "friends." I am not in the mood for chit chat given how fat and gross I feel.

The first spin class is great. I feel like I could go forever, and I am really into the music and everything else happening. However, the second is pure torture. Why didn't I drink more water??? I drank too much coffee and with no breakfast (the French toast bites don't count, right?), my mind easily wanders. It is eventually over, and I don't feel as disgusting, I do not look at myself in any of the mirrors in the gym locker room as I change and head out.

I am starving, and I pound a giant bottle of water on the drive to the supermarket. I walk into the store and grab a basket, since I'm only here to pick up a few things. On my way to the rotisserie chicken, I pass the bakery and throw in a baguette. I start eating it as I walk to the prepared food aisle. I grab a few more odds and ends and go by the candy aisle, where I notice they are having a sale on licorice. I pick up a 20-ounce Diet Coke and start to drink it as I wander on through the candy and cookie aisle. I glance and note the duality of my basket. Protein and low-carb vegetables on one side, sugar and processed food on the other. Whatever, my head is killing me. I go to the self-check-out line to avoid having to talk to an overly peppy clerk and get in my car. I tear open the licorice with my teeth and end up eating the entire bag by the time I get back to my house. I throw the empty bag away in the garbage cans under the recycling, pick up a Diet Coke from the garage fridge, and bring the rest of the groceries inside, where I make small talk with the sitter.

I am not sure whether to have the chicken for lunch or to not bother, since I had so much licorice in the car. I decide to think about it after I take a shower. I don't have a decision by the time I get back downstairs, but I do know I want to be alone so I can eat in privacy. I send the sitter home early with the excuse that the baby is asleep. I end up eating random processed kids' food after she leaves. I lie down, since I am so freaking exhausted from last night's sugar, the double spin class, the post-caffeine let-down, and my life.

When my two-year-old wakes up, we go to get my daughter from school. I glance at myself in the rearview mirror. My chin will not clear up. It is so annoying. I have worse skin now than when I was 15. The dermatologist gives me a different face wash every time I see her. If my skin doesn't get better by the next visit, there is talk of putting me on oral medication. I really do not want to go on it, but discussing zits and freckles at the same visit seems crazy to me.

I see my daughter at pickup. She is so cute, until she gets in the car snarling over not being picked line leader. I remind her today is Tuesday, so it is time for ballet and music class. Neither kid wants to go to either.

Thankfully, I have a large Diet Coke in my car and a bag of Jelly Bellies in the console. I take handfuls of the candy and put them in my lap, so the kids cannot see. The kids are so noisy in the back seat on the drive home, and traffic is awful. The candy bag is gone, and the Diet Coke is empty. I pull in the garage and think, "Oh no, dinner!" The kids are going to want to eat. I reach for the chicken and am grateful it will serve some purpose. I can't even look at food, but I throw together dinner for the kids. I somehow get through feeding and bathing them. My head is killing me again, but if I am ever going to get to sleep tonight, I cannot have any more caffeine. My husband texts me that he is stuck at work and won't be home until way past the kids' bedtime. I put them both to bed. My daughter is especially difficult tonight, as she wants to discuss why her dad isn't home yet and how come Christmas cannot be every day. I try really hard to not lose any remaining patience with her. Ugh! I want some time to myself.

I check my phone and I notice an annoying email from a woman I volunteer with at school. She is such a one-upper, makes me insane! If I am going to eat something before I go to bed, I have do it now. Who was I supposed to call this morning? What did my husband want me to do for him? Crap, I wish I could remember. Maybe we have ice cream left over from the other day....

That was how I lived forever, or so it seemed. If I was so smart, and had the family, the house, the husband, the things I thought would make me happy and content, why could I not lose the extra ten pounds? Why did I have secret stashes of candy? Same with the brain fog, given the baby was now two and sleeping through the night and still I couldn't remember anything for long. Acne became a constant issue in my thirties, which everyone from the doctor to the ladies at the makeup counter told me was either hormonal or I just needed a magic cream. I had low levels of depression, and I rationalized it by telling myself that everyone with small kids is tired. Wanting to nap all afternoon and stay up all night to eat in peace is perfectly acceptable.

This probably sounds familiar to you. If you are like me, you didn't see the forest for the trees. I was unable to see the relationship between what I was putting in my mouth and my energy levels. No matter how noble my intentions were, every Monday morning when I would start my newest diet or when I would do my walk of shame back in Weight Watchers, I somehow couldn't stay on my damn diet. Was I weak-willed? Why did it seem like so many other people could do it? Why could I do it when I was younger? Maybe the answer was to eat less. Or to only eat orange food. Or only fat. Or only dairy, or only watermelon, or whatever some D-list celebrity told me.

Looking back on it, I was not suffering from a lack of morals nor was my life insufficient in some major way. I was on a constant sugar roller coaster that I couldn't get off of. I had the best of intentions, but I couldn't kick the habit. Even when I managed to go sugar-free for a while, I couldn't maintain it. I wanted a life without stashes of candy or hiding wrappers, but I could not get there.

Once I did figure it out, I wanted to help other people, which I have been doing in my own coaching practice. However, I wanted to reach more women, and that is why I wrote this book. I wanted to help YOU. I know how you are feeling: the frustration, the annoying obsession with what's for lunch while struggling to be perfect, the "screw-its" that come on around 4 pm, and the swan dives into a jar of Nutella. I knew there had to be a better way, and that if I could find it and stay with it, I would share it with the world.

You, my dear friend, are getting the benefit of my years of green drinks, master cleanses, challenge groups, rice cakes, and two-point bars. Now that I know better, we will both do better. All you have to do is take my hand, and we will do this together.

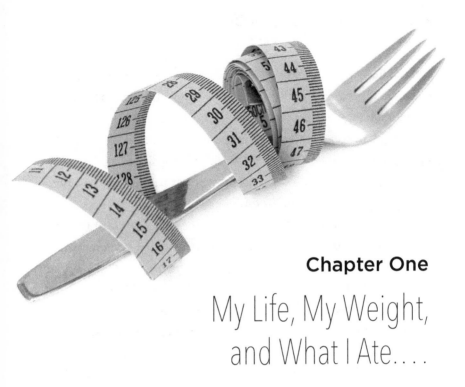

Chapter One

My Life, My Weight, and What I Ate....

ONE OF MY MOTHER'S FAVORITE MEMORIES of me as a toddler in the 1970s involved me and a giant red licorice rope. She would give me one in my umbrella stroller, I would gnaw on it, and she could get all of her shopping done at the mall in relative peace. I hear this story now and cringe.

However, I do use it as an example for my coaching clients and workshop participants to drive home the point that as a small child, I was given a powerful substance by my parent, and that I liked it enough to be quiet for a considerable amount of time. I was always super chatty. If we substituted heroin for licorice in the story, everyone would be horrified, right? But sugar is eight times more addictive, and the hardest addiction to kick. Why? Some of it is because it's so readily available –

you can find sugary snacks at every grocery store, convenience store, and office supply chain across the land. But mostly, it's because, as researchers have found, sugar is more addictive than cocaine.

I have struggled with body image problems since what feels like forever, but is at least junior high. I felt "fat" in the sixth grade, and I cannot remember a time since when I was not painfully aware of how much space I was taking up, and where I could find some sugar.

In the 90s, fat-free was the rage. It was also my personal heaven. I had decided to focus my obsession on licorice and gummies, anything chewy and fat-free. The beauty of fat-free, high-fructose corn syrup, AKA sugar, is that it hits your blood sugar like a ton of bricks. You can't stop eating it even if you wanted to, it is engineered to screw with your brain in just this way. Same things happen to kids who love soda, but I wasn't a soda kid, not a traditional sugary soda kid. I drank Diet Coke.

Around this same time, I decided I'd had enough of my childhood baby fat, and wanted to be skinny. It was the beginning of my weight obsession. Over the summer between ninth and tenth grade, I dropped thirty pounds. Yep, and I am 5'7. Teachers thought I had transferred in from a new school! I loved the attention, and the boys who had previously ignored me were suddenly interested. It was fantastic! However, I had to maintain the weight loss, right? So I did what every self-respecting girl does: find a way to have it all, through tons of exercise and/or flat-out bulimia.

At college, I would have periods when I would be "good" and not binge or engage in any crazy behaviors. Then I would be pretty "bad." I would stop by a grocery store after my shift at work and buy bags of gummy bears. I used tons of sweetener in coffee and drank diet soda by the gallon. My weight slowly crept up. My old way of keeping up with my eating by over-exercising, taking laxatives, and purging was not working anymore, but at the time, I blamed my weight gain on birth control, not on my eating habits

In grad school, I met the guy who would become my husband, and we went out to dinner all the time. I gained a good ten pounds in graduate school, which put me officially past the weight marker I had set back in high school with my baby fat. I didn't purge much then, but I sure binged a lot.

I moved to Chicago, where my then boyfriend was accepted into business school, in the dead of winter. I pretty much hid out in a giant puffy coat that resembled a duvet with arms when I left the apartment, which was next to never. After a particularly uncomfortable experience that spring as a friend's bridesmaid, I decided enough was enough: I was losing the weight. I lost 35 pounds, but never gave up sugar, nor did anyone say I was supposed to. This was when Weight Watchers was OK with whatever you wanted to eat, as long as it had some fiber shoved into it. It was a fabulous work-around as far as I was concerned. I will admit I felt good that I was able to maintain my weight loss and adhere to the plan. It was empowering to have such a sense of control and I loved the results. The compliments didn't hurt.

My husband and I got married, I was thin, and life was good. He worked 80-100 hours a week, and I worked out a ton. It never occurred to me to wonder why I still had acne, why I was so moody, or why I "had" to have something sweet by a certain time each day. I didn't connect the dots to understand why my weight was slowly creeping up again.

I got pregnant, and, for the first time in my life, immediately became the poster girl for perfect chemical-free eating. I was able to drink unsweetened iced tea! I wanted to be healthy for the baby. But once my daughter was born, I found staying home with a baby in the winter depressing, boring, and a lot of other things that threw me right back into my screwy eating habits. I still worked out and was somewhat "good," but working out wasn't enough of a counter-balance with being home all day with a three-month-old while my husband was working

18-hour days to keep me sane. Oh, that, and I didn't think I had a problem. I was still BFFs with denial.

It was after we moved to the NYC suburbs that I became an exercise teacher. I started with spinning. I needed to connect with grown-ups and had always liked working out, so I figured, why not? My son was born in February of 2009. Once the arsenal of family members who'd come to help out went back home, I got back on the coffee with sweetener, Diet Coke, and candy – my trifecta from hell.

I slowly gained a good ten pounds from where I wanted to be post-baby weight, and was always dieting. Granted, I wasn't visibly overweight or anywhere near being unreliable as an example when teaching. However, I wasn't happy with my body, and believed I could be if only I could stick to my freaking diet! Why couldn't I do it like other times?

Next came my yoga certification, and yet I still didn't lose enough weight for good with it. So much for inner peace. Then Pilates, but it, too, wasn't the magic exercise that would change the number on the scale or the one on the back of my jeans. Barre and TRX were great, but the scale didn't budge. I had the sugar trifecta working against me.

Then came the exercise shakes, which still make me cringe. None of it really worked for long. When I was doing the packaged shakes, we would have challenge groups where a bunch of women would support each other via Facebook to get healthy. I lost track of how many I did. Or how many times I lost the same five pounds in the three-week timespan of the group. Each and every time, we would be asked in the getting to know you stage "Why are you here?" I always wrote "I want to stop the food drama." Not sure if anyone realized what I was saying. I know I didn't really understand it at the time.

I finally do understand what I meant by *the food drama*. I was so flipping tired of the constant internal dialogue related to my weight and food. Was I being good or bad? Were my jeans going to fit today? Could

I lose enough weight fast enough that no one would know what I ate last night? Does this sound familiar to you? Have you also been aware of your weight, your size, and your daily calorie intake since forever? I bet you are pretty tired from it. I know I was.

I wanted someone to help me escape from this whole nightmare. I was hoping I would find the magic solution, pill, diet, or blog. It would have been amazing if my dream of being done with the ups and downs could be reality. Think of the extra room in my brain I would have if I wasn't constantly obsessing over: my body, if I look fat, how I feel fat, and what I want to eat next. I wanted it to stop for once and for all. I tried to find the magic pill, wand, or spell to make it stop. I have a pretty good feeling that you have as well. I bet you have been asking yourself why you can't stick to your diet too. Why does it have to be so stinking hard to live life and not be constantly thinking of weight and calories?

When I finally figured out what worked, I knew I had to share it with other women. Not just the ones I knew from school, or the ones who belong to my secret Facebook group, but all the women I could find. I wanted to help them, because I wish someone had helped me years ago. Think of how much sooner I could have lived free from the food drama if only I knew better.

I know the woman who struggles with sugar. I was her. I had to write a book for her. What would have helped me? What author would I have loved to run across at an airport bookstore on my way to a yoga retreat?

I would have wanted to know who she was, why she felt qualified to help me, if she had even helped herself, if it had lasted, and most: When could we start?

So let's get on with it already.

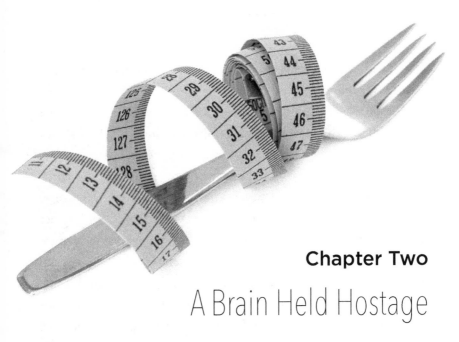

Chapter Two

A Brain Held Hostage

Erin, I never understood how food truly worked until you explained it in terms I could understand.
- Kelly, 42, lost 9.2 lbs in 3 weeks

WHEN I WAS A KID, there was a commercial to tell us kids to not do drugs. It had a sizzling frying pan, and the voiceover said "This is your brain." Then an egg would be cracked on the side of the frying pan and the voice would say "This is your brain on drugs." The eggs would cook up in about 15 seconds and then the screen would flash to a "don't do drugs" statement. I like to use the same idea with sugar. When my brain was on sugar, it was equally as fried as those stinking eggs.

In the food addiction world, we like to use the term "hijacked." It is a rather strong word nowadays, but give me some time to explain the reasoning. When we are being held hostage by sugar, we are impaired.

We cannot make independent decisions on what is in our best interests for our health or our bodies.

The introduction of high-fructose corn syrup (HFCS) into the modern diet only complicates the hijacked situation. HFCS was genetically modified to make us crave if we stop eating it.

Growing up in the 1970s, I aspired to be Wonder Woman, the mirror image of the Lynda Carter version from the show. I had the Underoos, the golden bracelets, even the action figures. The thing with Wonder Woman is she doesn't have a mortal enemy or anything she cannot conquer as she is perfect in every way, like any good Feminist icon. However, I can relate to a different member of the Justice League because I have learned I have something in common with Superman. I was not born light years away and sent to Earth as an infant; however, there is a substance I cannot tolerate – it is my weakness or my kryptonite. It is high-fructose corn syrup (HFCS). It is the main ingredient in licorice. It makes me want to eat it once it is out of my system, because the little genetic markers are lying in my fat cells demanding to be fed.

Artificial Isn't Any Better

One of my favorite things to do was to go to the movies with my kids and eat candy, popcorn, and get a massive Diet Coke. I mean one the size of a swimming pool. It would usually send me into a giant sugar tailspin later on in the day, but at the time, I didn't care. I was under the Halo Effect. Simply put, anything with implied health benefits such as a diet soda or sugar-free gives the consumer implied permission to eat more later since they were so healthy in their earlier choices.

Now we are learning artificial sweeteners make us crave sugary foods more than sugar. Simply put, they let our brain think that something sweet is coming into our bodies by turning on the receptors of the pleasure centers of our brain. When the sugary food doesn't come, the cravings get stronger, and we end up eating more sugar.

Why Is This Worth the Hassle?

The pain of not changing needs to be greater than the pain of the
sacrifice required for change.
- Tony Robbins

Let's face it, I could have been on the sugar roller coaster for longer. It wouldn't have been pretty, and eventually my body would have started to break down even further. I was able to change my life and my body, and my outlook.

I have lost my cravings, the extra weight, the brain fog, and the lack of energy. I did this without surgery or by running away from home and joining an ashram. If I can do it, I know you can.

The current Standard American Diet (SAD) is one of very little vegetables, lots of meat, processed food, and sugar. It is essentially high-calorie malnutrition. The current SAD is linked to diabetes, heart disease, and cancer.

Sugar comes in many forms. The obvious ones are fruit, then sugars from turbinado (less processed) to what we would all recognize as white table sugar. The other 48 names include dextrose, brown sugar, cane crystals, cane sugar, corn sweetener, corn syrup, corn syrup solids, crystal dextrose, evaporated cane juice, fructose sweetener, fruit juice sweetener. For avid label readers, we might be avoiding an obvious word such as sugar but would we walk away from maltose in yogurt? Or rice syrup in packaged roast beef? Even if our minds do not register it, our bodies will, and our cravings will kick in causing havoc when all we had consumed was what seemed like an innocuous sandwich.

Our First Drug

Addiction experts often say abusers have their first sip of alcohol during their preteen years. Most of us had sugar before we were one. How often have we all seen the one-year-old birthday cake pictures? Popsicles in grade school and snow cones at the street fair.

Using the addiction analogy, those of us that are sugar-sensitive often have learned to associate sweetness with good feelings, with happiness and celebration. Society doesn't help with the cooking channels and the recipe exchanges. It is Christmas, so let's have Grandma's special cake! You got straight As, so we are taking you out for ice cream. The hotel you are staying in is welcoming you to the room, so here, have some cookies! Sugar is love. Sugar is comfort. Sugar is your friend. Sugar is a party in a bag, or a waxed cup, or an ice cream container. Sugar is everything and everywhere!

Once sugar is introduced into our lives, there is no turning back. I can still remember how happy my daughter was when she stole my iced coffee full of artificial sweetener at two. I would have to wrestle it away from her chubby little toddler arms. Thankfully, she finds them gross now at eleven and hates most sweet things.

Are You Impacted?

Women seem to love to say to me things like, "Hey Erin, I am a total sugar addict," in a wellness workshop. Or I'll meet a mother at a coffee shop who says "I need to go to Sugar Anonymous, *haha,*" while downing a large Unicorn Frappuccino at 2 pm. I just got a text while writing this: "I am back from Summer Vacation. I gained 14 pounds. Now what? LOL." I try to take these comments in a good way as they keep me employed and at least these things are being discussed openly. When I was truly suffering, I was not making jokes about it. I was too food hungover to make jokes and too embarrassed to text an acquaintance about it.

Two cool additional things happened in my search to fix myself: 1) I became super knowledgeable as to what the hell had happened to me; 2) I became obsessed with the idea of helping others to get off of it as well. Wouldn't it have been fantastic if someone like me had been around to help me back when I was the old me? So old me, come and find the new me already!

If the future me could have come back and said just one thing to the present me, it would have been to pay attention to the white stuff. Meaning sugar, flour, and artificial sweeteners. I started to notice through my food journaling, that those three things would always mess me up. The less of them I ate, the more success I would have in maintaining my weight and in weight loss. Simply put, the less white stuff I ate, the better.

I have spent a lot of time studying food addiction, listening to some of the best researchers on the planet discuss super high-level terms that only nutrition nerds like me care about. (The nutrition nerd stuff is coming later on, but you will have to wait.) They lecture a lot about brain chemistry, and they have shown me in-depth addiction models, and have gone into great detail on relapse prevention.

Amongst the Food Addiction Field, there is an agreed upon spectrum and your spot on the chart might change depending on your life and what foods you are consuming on a regular basis. There have been times when I was eating the frosting off my kid's birthday cake when everyone was in bed versus today when the cake would be safe in the house. Generally, I do very well on a Sugar Dependency Test. In my typical overachiever fashion, I usually get an A! However, that doesn't mean my grade has not severely plummeted on occasion since I figured it out. Your grade will rise and fall too, but for now, let's ask ourselves a few questions.

These questions have been borrowed from Overeaters Anonymous. Don't worry, there is a method too my madness. I adapted these from

OA, because in only a few questions, a great deal can be assessed. The reason why we are doing this is not to scare you or to try to persuade you that you need to go to a twelve-step food group.

1. Do I go on food binges for no apparent reason, sometimes eating until I'm stuffed or even feel sick?
2. Do I have feelings of guilt, shame, or embarrassment about my weight or the way I eat?
3. Do I eat sensibly in front of others, or not at all, and then make up for it when I am alone?
4. When my emotions are intense, whether positive or negative, do I find myself reaching for food?
5. Do I fantasize about how much better life would be if I had a handle on my food?

Have you answered "yes" to several of these questions? If so, it is possible that you have, or are well on your way to having, a problem.

Now I borrowed and revised this list for those of us who cannot stick to a diet. You do not have to circle "Yes" on every one of these questions to know you might have a problem sticking to a diet. Looking back upon my life, I knew I was not like everyone else when it came to food – not that I was equipped to do anything about it, when I was about eight.

If you opened up this book, if you bought this book, if you downloaded this book, odds are you know you might have an issue with white stuff. If you have tried 1000 times to stick to your diet, you have "failed" on 999 diets, or you have started 1000 diets only to gain weight, you might have an issue with white stuff. If you wish you ate less white stuff, but can't manage to get through an entire day without it, you probably have an issue with white stuff. If you have spent a great deal of time trying to get rid of white stuff in your diet, only to not be able to do it, you probably have an issue with sugar, flour, and/or artificial sweetener.

Did I ever go on sugar binges for no apparent reason? Of course! Maybe it was a Tuesday, or I needed it. Once I had a little hidden sucrose in my yogurt, next thing I knew I had eaten an entire family-size pack of Skittles in a darkened movie theater. I remember eating a giant bowl of green grapes when I was around twelve, without even realizing it, because I was watching TV.

I go way back with guilt, shame and embarrassment with my weight. I can tell you how much I weighed in the 8th grade, the 9th grade, the 10th grade, when I started college, when I started Weight Watchers, when I graduated from Weight Watchers, when I had a baby, three days after I had the seven-pound baby (BTW, I had only lost two pounds), two weeks after I had the baby (down 25 pounds thankfully), and on and on. I have avoided going to the doctor the time I was pretty sure I had a sinus infection over the fear of being weighed. I was a little relived when I moved out of Hawaii based on their driver's licenses listing bodyweight. Seriously, who wants to live anywhere but Hawaii? Uh, on my list of pros for leaving was the driver's license. Who was I kidding? That whole line of thinking was really about sugar.

Eating sensibly in front of others and making up for it when I was alone was my favorite thing to do. I was always a salad-dressing-on-the-side person, but I had candy in the car for the drive home. Passing on dessert in the restaurant and having hot water with lemon while everyone else ordered was acceptable to me, but once I got home, all bets were off. I would buy my kids candy for a holiday, and they would pick at it. Through the grace of God, neither of my kids give a crap about sugar. It is rather amazing. After a few days of trying to not tear into it in front of them, I would declare it time to give it away to the soldiers. Which I would eventually, once I had picked out what I needed. Now let's circle back to my shame and guilt.

Intense emotions would lead me eventually to sugar. When I am super-stressed, I am not hungry. I know that is a rarity in some circles. The super-stressed phase can last a day or months, depending on the stressor. Once things calm down, almost like a way for my system to relax, I would go for the sugar, and I would go hard. A few years ago, something major happened in my personal life, which led me to finally putting sugar behind me. I was under intense stress for weeks; when I look back at the pictures, I had dropped too much weight, too quickly. It was not cute. Since everyone has smartphones out constantly, I can also track when I stopped feeling numb by all the documentation. When I was coming out of my numb phase, I remember eating nothing but candy one day over the holidays. The intense emotions I was finally feeling were unbearable, so I went and hid in a box of toffee.

My favorite question of the big five is the last one, "Did I ever fantasize about how life would be if I had a handle on my sugar?" Abso-freakin-lutely! Those were my hobbies: fantasizing about quitting sugar and eating it, of course. It would have been a gift from heaven or a dream come true if I woke up one morning, with none of the physical, emotional, and psychological consequences of sugar. I had fantasies where such things happened. Where there would be a magical diet, or pill, or hell, a fairy godmother would grant me clemency from this prison. However, she never showed up. So I had to save myself.

Here is where I come in for you. I am your fairy godmother/Glinda, the Good Witch of the North. I prefer to think of myself like Helen Bonham Carter in the recent version of *Cinderella*, with a great blond wig, biting wit, and a phenomenal dress. Not a huge fan of Glinda from *Wicked* – she was a tad self-absorbed, but you get my point. However, I do not believe in simply granting you a magical cure, because much like Cinderella lost her stagecoach, you would be back in the white stuff once the clock strikes midnight. With something this deep, you need to do the work; a quick fix will not take. I will grant you a clear path to life out of the white stuff. All you have to do is meet me halfway and we will get there together.

In this book you will learn:

- Why diets are so hard to stick to
- What is preventing us from sticking to our diets
- How I learned to stick to my diet by not being on one
- Living the rest of your life without a diet, yet maintaining your weight loss
- How to combat any food obstacle
- To ditch the diet mentality for good

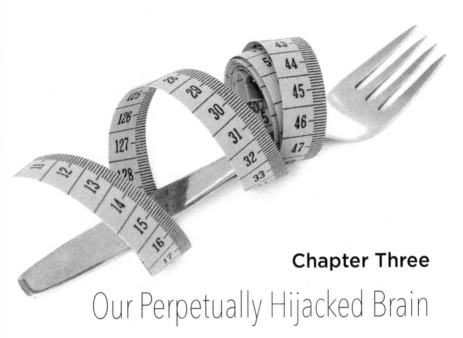

Chapter Three

Our Perpetually Hijacked Brain

Not everyone would know intellectually what needs to be done to get
from here to there - they would just know there is a problem. I believe
your book will help solve the problem for women.
- Monica, age 52, lost 12 lbs in 7 weeks

ONCE UPON A TIME, humans did not have processed or refined carbohydrates in our diet. We lived off of protein and fruits and vegetables. There were not any Twinkies or Frappucinos. Our bodies would have to convert protein, fruit and vegetables to sugar for our brain to think. Then refined carbohydrates or processed carbohydrates were introduced in all forms. It doesn't take much time or effort at all for our body to absorb the sugar from the food as the work has already been done for the body before it is eaten, in the processing. This changed the brain dramatically. We liked carbohydrates. It was great, at first.

It meant something fun was going on – we were celebrating. The first couple of seconds of sugar and flour makes our entire body happy. Our dopamine receptors were made happy, mimicking the effect of mind-altering drugs such as cocaine.

From this point on in the book, I am going to use the term sugar to include white sugar and flour. The reason is our brains. Modern wheat and grains have "been genetically altered to provide processed food manufacturers the greatest yield at the lowest cost; consequently, this once benign grain has been transformed into a nutritionally empty ingredient which causes blood sugar to spike more rapidly than eating pure table sugar and has addictive properties that cause hunger, overeating, and fatigue." The Diet Doctor, Dr. William Morris, in *Wheat Belly*.

To our brains and our bodies, table sugar and white flour are not very different; they are both digested and metabolized essentially as sugar, as they are already processed before being consumed. If you have a problem with one, you will eventually have a problem with the other. Every so often, I will have a client who swears she is the exception to the rule. She will freely admit she cannot be anywhere near a breadbasket or pizza, but cake is fine. Cake might have been fine when she was having a great deal of wheat and grains, but once those are eliminated, she could very well find herself going for sugar. The cake that was not a problem could now be. So all sugar needs to be out.

When we attempt to pull back on sugar, our brain is not happy. The chemicals in our brain are not happy, our mood is not happy, our body is not happy. To put it bluntly, it is as if we are negotiating with terrorists, but the terrorists are in our head.

Sugar Demands More Sugar

Many studies of sugar involve rats. I find it fascinating how rats mimic humans in similar situations. For example, when rats become addicted to cocaine, they will forgo rat food to have cocaine. Then the same rats are offered high-fructose corn syrup (HFCS). This newer type of sugar (HFCS) was created in a lab to be more efficiently addictive and cheaper to mass produce. It is commonly seen in things like candy corn or used in soda. Our cocaine-addicted rats preferred the HFCS to cocaine. Even when the rats started to go into withdrawal from the cocaine, the rats went to the HFCS, implying they were more addicted to the HFCS.

Our beloved HFCS rats also taught us another important lesson about sugar. The rats needed more and more sugar to have the same result. So, their sugar dependence was progressive. The level of HFCS that was sufficient for them not go into withdrawal last week, wasn't enough this week.

So what do lab rats have to do with us? First of all, it illustrates how dangerous of a substance sugar is. It is not a matter of willpower or being a good person. Rats are not moral or immoral, they are simply responding to the chemicals in the substances they prefer. They responded to the chemical in cocaine, and preferred HFCS to cocaine. Think about that one. The chemical in your average soda is more addictive than an illegal street drug – a drug that to the average person is the most addictive substance in existence. This shows why it is so stinking difficult to stop going by Starbucks at 10 a.m. or why, no matter how hard you try, every day at 4 p.m. you are into the jelly beans at work.

If we were to take away all of the social constructs around sugar, all of the warm and fuzzy memories with Grandma making cakes, and cooking shows of bake-offs, and simply look at sugar as a chemical, it would be easier to see that sugar is addictive, nutritionally void, and dangerous. It has been linked to obesity, diabetes, cavities, insatiable hunger, and even cognitive decline. I am not advocating banning bananas; I am taking the emotion out of it and looking at the chemical makeup of sugar and what the logical conclusion would be if it were introduced to us now.

I recently spoke to a leading expert in the war against sugar. He feels in 20 or 30 years, we will look back at how we are currently eating sugar with the same disgust with which we now view cigarette smoking. What was once commonplace is now considered unhealthy and downright unacceptable by the average person. It is common knowledge that cigarette smoking is dangerous and will lead to an early death. We no longer have smoking sections in planes, restaurants, or bars. Cigarettes are banned on public streets in many parts of the country. Small children know cigarettes will kill you and the labeling on every type of cigarette package is extremely graphic. A small minority of people still choose to smoke, which is their choice. However, the average person is aware of the dangers of smoking and each year, fewer people in America smoke than the year before.

Secondly, the progressive need of the rats to have more and more HFCS is crucial to understand. Have you found that a small mocha was enough for you to get through your morning but it has now morphed into the grande mocha plus a scone? The sugar crutch will only get worse. It will not plateau. I am not trying to scare you, but to be honest about the science. I had to understand the chemical nature of what was going on with me and solve that, before I could tackle the emotional and psychological habit of sugar.

Women and Sugar

Women are biochemically susceptible to sugar due to our monthly cycle. Yep, we are biologically hardwired to want sugary carbs after ovulation but before menstruation. PMS is not an urban legend, or an excuse to run out and find the biggest carton of ice cream at the grocery store. It is science.

Last spring, I went to a fundraiser for an eating disorder prevention non-profit. Dr. Kelly Klump, of Michigan State University, conducted a study on college-aged women who had already been self-diagnosed as having binge eating episodes. She concluded that there is a strong correlation between the combined oral contraceptive birth control pill and binges; it increased the frequency of their episodes. Now, remember the pill mimics the natural hormones so a woman doesn't get pregnant. The super-smart scientist did things like putting one identical twin on the pill and not the other to see what would happen and such. Long story short, the more progesterone, the more likely they were to binge in the time period when progesterone was highest – in a nutshell, when PMS hits. I know this isn't breaking news to most of us, but knowing the science behind what the hell I had been going through helped me stop shaming myself and look for a solution that stuck. I found a solution in science.

Caffeine/Fake Sugar Conundrum

My first real experience with any type of coffee was in high school. My BFF and I were hanging around a little coffee house so she could flirt with the barista. I remember ordering some sort of raspberry coffee-like concoction with a lot of whipped cream. The cute barista didn't charge us, as he was flirting back. After I drank it, I asked the barista what was in it. He told me in great detail how I basically ordered an artificially flavored milkshake with a splash of coffee.

I used to have a big problem with coffee. I didn't know how to make it palatable. When I got to college, I decided I needed to drink it like a real grown-up – or at least the ones I saw in the movie *Singles*. I was so conflicted, as I wanted to add tons of whole milk and sugar, to basically drink defrosted mocha ice cream. Since I was on a diet my entire life and was still annoyed at the raspberry mocha incident from above, I would add skim milk and a lot of Equal. So it tasted like watery nothing, but I kept drinking away. Now I know the caffeine/artificial sweetener combo, similar to the one in diet soda, creates havoc on our hormones and makes our sugar cravings intensify. So, then we want to eat more sugar, which defeats the purpose of consuming the artificial sweetener in the first place, right?

Artificial sweeteners have been described as sugar methadone. A substitute to get you off the hard drug, but not a solution to the addiction at hand. So I can buy sugar methadone at my local Stop N Shop and that is A-OK with everyone?!? Let's put the whole government regulation issue on the shelf for a while and get back to why artificial sweeteners need to be dumped along with sugar. They keep us in the sugar cycle. It might seem like a short-term solution, but I needed a clean break from the whole scene.

Like a Gummy Frog in a Pot

There is a story about a frog in a pot of water. If you turn up the water slowly enough, the frog will not notice he is sitting in boiling water until it is too late to jump out, because, well, he will be, you know, dead. This is what I think of when it comes to my sugar story. (Only my frog would be a gummy one – which can't be boiled because it would break down, but that is not my point, now is it!) Now that I am off of sugar, I can look back and realize all the slow changes that were not due to age, or hormones, or life, but due to excessive sugar.

I was one moody bitch. It was due to the weather, the kids fighting, or my husband breathing. I do not remember being happy on Tuesday and blah on Wednesday. However, mild depression and mood swings are associated with excessive sugar consumption. Don't get me wrong, the weather still can suck, my kids will fight over nothing, and my husband still snores. The difference is I do not wake up snarling at everyone about it.

The gut is the new black! No, seriously, it is. No one used to ever talk about their gut flora or their biome, except for my colon therapist, Kelly. She was the only person I talked to about it, because let's face it, no one really wants to talk about those things. No matter how many times I read *Everybody Poops* to my kids, did it ever make it OK to discuss such things with anyone but my colon hydrotherapist? I did learn many things during my years with Kelly; mostly her life story but a lot about our internal plumbing, and this was way before it was cool. The majority of our immune system is in our intestinal tract.

You know what our GI tract cannot have if we want to keep the good bacteria happy and the bad ones away? Sugar. You know what I was feeding them forever? That's right, sugar. I would be doubled over in pain with Kelly after every single stinking holiday. Post Easter and Halloween were always especially brutal. I won't get any more graphic. Let's just say those issues are gone as well.

My skin as a teenager was good. I had the occasional zit. Nothing major. I look at pictures of myself from high school and college, and I might have the occasional little blemish, but nothing noteworthy. My skin got progressively worse starting in grad school, and by the time I could afford a dermatologist in my late 20s, I was dealing with cystic acne. I was told it was due to hormones at my age, and it happens to many women. I had to go on oral meds and get breakouts injected with cortisone because they hurt so stinking bad, I couldn't wait for them to work themselves out. Never mind going around the world with a giant zit and a baby on your hip like something out of MTV's *Teen Mom*. I was going to one of the best dermatologists in NYC and given tons of creams and medications. I was never asked about my sugar, wheat, or artificial sweetener consumption. Now I know sugar increases inflammation in the body overall, it increases blood sugar, and confuses the heck out of your hormones resulting in acne. Post sugar breakup, my skin is good. I still obsess over premature aging and wish Botox grew on trees, but the constant zits have gone the way of the Sweet Tarts – as in, out of my life.

One of my favorite parts of *The Wizard of Oz* has always been when everything goes from black and white to color when Dorothy and Toto land on the Wicked Witch of the West. That is the best way I can describe how things taste now that I have stopped deadening my taste buds with sugar. Everything tastes better without the constant bombardment of chemicals. Things smell better – or worse, in some instances. My taste buds took at least a month to wake back up from the sugar coma I put them in. Yours will too, just be patient. As a warning, some things might taste or smell flat-out disgusting once you ditch all the sugars. I remember smelling a fellow passenger opening up a bag of Blue Chips on an airplane and just about gagging. I used to love them.

I had a really annoying 12 pounds I could not lose. Nothing that ruined my health, not enough that I would be deemed, you know, overweight, but enough that it shook my self-confidence. I have been teaching Spin, Pilates, and Yoga for ten years, so to have any extra weight was not cool. In addition, with my body type, which is called an inverted triangle, it is even worse. It consists of broad shoulders (thanks Dad), small waist, and narrow hips at 5'7. So if I am at my current fighting weight, it can all work. If I have extra pounds, it goes to my face almost immediately, my upper arms, and to my muffin top. It isn't a cute distribution like a Kardashian who gets a bigger butt and everyone gives her a high five for loving herself. I was asked if I was expecting when I went with a pregnant friend to a maternity store (true story) when I was a little heavier.

So, these extra pounds were really bothering me, but I could not lose them for good. They kept finding me! I would drop a few for a while, and they would come back with friends. It was an annoying dance I wanted no part of, and yet I could not get off the dance floor. Once I got rid of sugar, the twelve pounds left for good and took another four with them. I went down three pants sizes and started buying bikinis again at 40. I got my groove back, and you will too.

A Brief History of Sugar

Every once in a while, I get a very change-resistant client who likes to tell me how sugar is natural because they can find the organic version at Whole Foods, so I need to give it a rest and leave them and their giant piña colada alone. I disagree on many levels, one of which is what our modern culture chose to do to sugar.

Where did it come from?

Let's start in the beginning, back in the BC days, when it is thought cane sugar developed in Polynesia and its use spread to India. In 510 BC, the Emperor Darius of Persia invaded India and discovered a plant that "gives us honey without the bees." This discovery was a closely guarded secret for centuries, as the finished product could be exported for a large profit.

Sugar was discovered by western Europeans as a result of the Crusades in the eleventh century AD. Crusaders returning home talked of this "new spice" and how pleasant it was. The first sugar was recorded in England in 1099. The subsequent centuries saw a major expansion of western European trade with the East, including the importation of sugar. When Columbus sailed to the Americas, he took sugar cane plants to grow in the "New World." The climate in the Caribbean was perfect for such a plant, and the growth of the sugar cane industry there began.

By 1750, there were 120 sugar refineries in Britain. Sugar was still a luxury and it was extremely lucrative, to the extent that sugar was known by some as "white gold." Governments saw an opportunity. England had a sugar tax for almost 100 years until the tax was done away with in 1874, making sugar finally accessible for the ordinary British citizen.

In the US, the average consumption per person was six pounds per person per year in the 1780s. The number increased as the sugar beet industry grew and as the US signed the 1876 Treaty with Hawaii. During Prohibition, soda surged in popularity. Americans never stopped drinking it, with or without rum. During WWII, sugar was rationed, starting in spring of 1942. Armies were burning or cutting off access to the cane fields in the Pacific, and the war effort needed sugar to make things such as antiseptics. Government files at the time urged housewives to sweeten cakes with syrup left over from canned fruit.

Once the war was over, sugar consumption increased, and now the average American consumes 130 pounds per year, most of it in the form of high fructose corn syrup. Sugar is now a large problem for the lowest rung on our economic ladder. Other additives that are commonly used today as a replacement for sugar are aspartame, cyclamate, saccharin, stevia, Sucralose, and a wide variety of naturally formed substitutes such as Brazzein, Thaumatin, Curculin, Monellin and others. Some of their perceived advantages are lack of calories (sweetened weight loss food), dental care, diabetes (sweetened food), cost, and other factors. This is highly debatable as artificial sweeteners may cause a chemical reaction in the brain to make the individual still crave sweets – and in fact, the average artificial sweetener user weighs more than the average real sugar user. So much for Diet Cokes!

Modern Day Sugars and Sweeteners

In the 20th century, sugars received large competition from artificial sweeteners and high-fructose corn syrup, which was developed by Richard O. Marshall and Earl P. Kooi in 1957. This product received several upgrades to its formula, and from 1977 its popularity rose greatly after United States raised sugar import taxes significantly. With abundance of locally produced corn, American manufacturers quickly developed sugar manufacturing plants, and introduced high-fructose corn syrup in various food products. Even internationally well-known products such as Coca-Cola and Pepsi use ordinary sugar in a majority of the countries, but in the United States they switched to high-fructose corn syrup.

Where is the government?

Remember when the British government saw an opportunity to tax sugar in the 1700s, and in the WWII era in America, the government felt it was OK to dictate how women prepared cakes in their own homes? Well, modern governments are still involved in our lives through sugar. However, the white sugar we see is nothing in comparison to the sugar we do not see in processed foods and drinks. The prices we pay for white sugar at the grocery store are only part of the underlying cost. The US government attempts to control the prices of commodities or goods while allowing for moderate volatility through subsidies.

Nonetheless, some parts of the US government acknowledge the obesity epidemic; however, other departments work with the sugar lobby (there is such a thing) to hide the truth. Want to guess which major companies donate to the sugar lobby? Coca-Cola and Heinz are among the main donors.

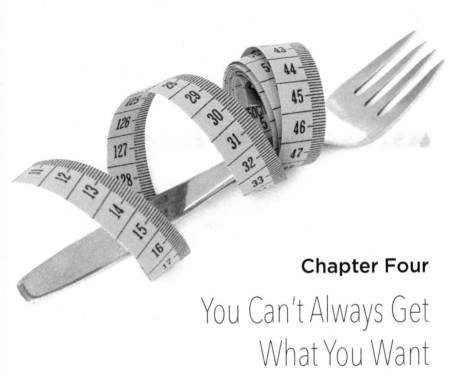

Chapter Four

You Can't Always Get What You Want

THE ROLLING STONES' classic song lyrics, "You can't always get what you want, but if you try sometimes you might find you get what you need," summarizes my theory on food, now that I have made it past sugar.

I am about to write a few positive things about sugar, but I want you to reserve judgment until the end of the chapter. So don't stop reading and tell yourself "Erin wrote sugar is great, so hand over the cupcakes." The first time we ate sugar and felt a chemical reaction to it, we did not realize we were signing up for symptoms such as premature aging, heart disease, depression, and tooth decay. Sugar can feel fantastic! Especially on a chemical level. On an emotional level, we often associate it with celebrations, love, and fun. Psychologically, it can be used to get us through the day, as an attempt to combat sleep deprivation, and a way to numb out.

Here is a simply way to explain what sugar does to our body. (Remember, sugar includes flour and artificial sweeteners.)

1. You eat or drink sugar
2. Your blood sugar rises, dopamine (a feel-good chemical) is released in the brain and insulin has to be secreted to handle the blood sugar spike
3. The high insulin causes immediate fat storage, and blood sugar dramatically plummets
4. Low blood sugar levels cause increased appetite and cravings for sugar. The body craves the lost sugar "high".

This is why it is such a bitch to walk away from. Addiction experts have told me sugar is the hardest substance to beat and the easiest to run back to. I would type that again, but you would think it was a typo, so let me express it a different way. Going off sugar is not an easy task. It isn't like Five Ways to Declutter Your Desk Drawer. You need to be committed to breaking up with sugar for good.

Would you look at your fairy godmother/Glinda and start to make excuses, rationalizations, or fake promises to her? Would you tell her how happy you are to see her, but to come back after the Super Bowl? Or a month before the high school reunion? Are you really willing to postpone the progress? Through your actions, you are saying the mood swings, the headaches, acne, hijacked brain, and bloating are worth the food. Now that I am offering you a way out, take it. Do not wait for the perfect time – there will never be one. I completely understand your hesitation, I was there time and time again, but this time is different because you have me. This time is unrelated to the others due to knowledge you have about your brain on sugar. This time will be independent of all the others because you have made up your mind that you are done with the food drama.

You will have to make some changes. However, didn't you ask for this to go away? Did you really think you could keep eating the Twix and ditch the brain fog? Hold onto the bread bowl and walk away from the acne? Let me walk you through why I had to make this choice and why I need you to as well.

The Myth of Moderation

We can all agree on the existence of feel-good myths in modern day culture. You know: The waitress who splits the winning lottery ticket with the cop since he didn't have cash for a tip and they win four million dollars, or the guy who sells his VW bus and starts Apple with a friend. These stories give us hope in humanity and make us want to keep on keeping on. When it comes to sugar, I found moderation a myth. I tried it in my post Weight Watchers years, and it did not work. I might not have gained my weight back, but I had every other horrible symptom in the book and was generally miserable.

Moderation told me a calorie is a calorie and I could eat whatever I wanted as long as it fit into my point allowance (daily calorie allotment). You are probably like me, and this did not work for you either. This type of thinking didn't work for me, as I would have fiber cookies sweetened with fruit juice for breakfast or sugared shredded wheat and nonfat milk plus fruit, tons of Diet Coke, eat high sugar/low fat, and be starving the rest of the day. I was always hungry after dinner. I could not close my kitchen three hours before bed like I can now. I remember eating tubs of Cool Whip with a spoon when my husband was working late, along with mint fat-free meringues. Now this always fit into my point allowance, but I was flipping nuts and always hungry.

Moderation would tell me I could have sugar in small doses, right? Well, my body doesn't respond to sugar like a normal person. I know this based upon years of beating my head against a wall. I have tried to just have a small piece of cake at my kids' birthday parties, and I would find myself hours later scraping all the frosting off of the leftover cake and eating it when everyone was in bed. Moderation didn't work for me. If you're here, reading this book, I'm guessing it hasn't worked for you, either.

I would eat only dessert for the annual BBQ we throw, figuring a calorie is a calorie and we were having a Ben and Jerry's sundae truck come to our house. This would result in me scarfing down my sundae plus my kids' leftover sundaes that had frozen into rock-hard globs in the freezer. High fives to moderation! One of my schemes involved me having candy only in the previews before the actual movie started. Well, I would start to panic that I wouldn't finish in time and then I would feel sick for the entirety of the movie from eating Junior Mints so quickly. Big love for moderation! There is some major bad blood between me and moderation!

Life with an Allergy

I have a good friend with celiac disease. To Brenda and her family, it is simply part of life. She has her own bread, her own snacks, and prepares her own foods. Brenda will call ahead when they go to a new restaurant to make sure she can get what she needs. With the airlines, Brenda has a standing requirement for a gluten-free meal. If some sort of gluten is somehow ingested, Brenda immediately gets sick and stays sick for days. Her body is rejecting it, and it is not cute or comfortable.

This is how I now view sugar and me. I am allergic to it. I know this not because of a medical test (which does not exist by the way), but because of how I react to sugar. You probably do not need a blood test to tell if you need to stay away from sugar. Even if I did not react to it badly, let's face it, who feels fabulous after a lot of sugar?? However, why do we do it? You probably have seen a specific class of magazines at the passport renewal office, car wash waiting areas, and the DMV. You know, the ones we would never buy or subscribe to but, if we are stuck there, will read. They almost always have some sort of bold statement and it will involve a number. The topics vary from "10 ways to make your Fourth-of-July Jell-O mold more exciting" to "10 tips to lose 5 lbs in 7 days." I wish they would educate the captive audience stuck in various waiting rooms about the symptoms of needing to drop sugar instead. They could educate us on why it is not OK to always be hungry after you eat, which I am sure you have experienced many times. The article needs to include why we still have acne, or mood swings, or bloat. The magazine needs to highlight why we find ourselves eating ice cream in the dark at night, or while driving the kids to ballet, or why the idea of giving up the 4 p.m. Diet Coke used to make me want to cry. This would make the annoying wait at the car wash a much better use of our time, don't you think?

Artificial sweetener or some variation of sugar is in chewing gum and most crackers and yogurt, or basically anything that comes in a package, container, or can. I try to avoid all types of sugars, since I crave it when I ingest even small amounts, even accidentally. Sugar creates the need for more sugar, and artificial sugar messes things up just as much. So, I had to stop eating anything in a package. Which can be a giant pain in the butt. I totally acknowledge it, but if you want to take back your life, isn't it worth a little extra legwork in the grocery store?

My Quest

I am a *Game of Thrones* fan. Not avid, as in I have a tattoo of Westeros on my back or anything, but I make a point of watching it and have been known to text about it while watching it with friends. I have read every book and have a strong opinion on the last couple of seasons since HBO ran out of original material. On the show, a main character has been gone from her home for six seasons, and she has changed a ton since she left. A lot has happened to her, and she has seen way too much. I am not implying or even joking that I am like Arya Stark who went on a quest and became a faceless assassin. However, I have been on a quest of sorts to figure out this sugar thing once and for all. I was so sick and tired of it all. The drama, the Monday-morning promises to myself, hiding candy wrappers, and having clothes in my closet I couldn't wear all the time. I had been wrestling with it for what felt like forever and I was done being on the losing team. So, like any heroine on a quest, I had to look far and wide.

So what exactly is a quest? According to my friend Google, "it is a long or strenuous search for something." I was looking to fix myself. It took a long time. I spent way too much time doing the sugar shuffle, and I do not want you doing it one more day – it sucks, let's face it. It sure was strenuous.

I did not know how to even start to get away from sugar as I had been told forever that low fat/high carb was the way to be healthy. I knew carbs were essentially processed as sugar by our bodies and I had been known to eat too much bread in a pinch. High carb/low fat was what everyone considered healthy when I was growing up, and who was I to argue with what "everyone" knew?

Thankfully, by this point in my life, I had learned a little bit about Paleo. I knew enough to know I did not want to call myself Paleo because people who are Paleo only want to talk about how they are Paleo and to attempt to convert you to being Paleo. That, and I gained weight on Paleo. It was due to all the dates and dipping chicken in crushed pistachios, and then frying it in coconut oil. Just because the cave people could have done it (assuming they had a Whole Foods to buy organic crushed pistachios from), didn't make it work for me, but that isn't my point.

I must have at least 50 or so diet/nutrition books in my house – just as many recipe books – and, I am sure, at least as many on my cloud. I have been on this quest longer than I thought when I really look back. I just wasn't looking in the right places, or asking the right questions to the right people.

I knew there were those who had ditched sugar permanently and still wanted to get out of bed in the morning. I just had to find them, and get them to tell me how to do it. Oh and it would be really great if the rest of the world adapted to my new regimen since I had decided enough was enough and didn't want to be tempted.

In my quest, I ended up becoming a Food Addiction Counselor, one of the first ever. I went to Iceland to finish the training, where I trained with experts from all over the world. I went to two different twelve-step food programs to listen, learn, and see how they were different from a diet club. Both are offshoots of Alcoholics Anonymous. Overeaters Anonymous (OA) is the one most people have heard of. I was expecting to hear something like the Weight Watchers meetings I had attended, and they weren't similar. We didn't have a leader, pay set dues, or get weighed in. Yes, the topic of food came up at OA but it was more of a symptom of the other areas of their lives. I heard members discuss their eating diagnosis, weight loss or gain, inability to be around buffets, or how mad they still were at their deceased parents. Some of the members of OA were considerably overweight, while you and I would consider others to be extremely underweight. They all identified as "compulsive overeaters," while others would also add terms such as "bulimarexic, recovering binge-eater, or over-exerciser."

I also attended Grey Sheet Anonymous (GSA) which came from OA. Members of GSA have a list of foods they are allowed to eat, period, end of discussion. Very strict meal times, portions, meeting attendance, and speaking with sponsors on a daily basis. GSA is a relatively new twelve-step program, and many people have found long-standing results from their program.

I read all the literature both programs had and a lot of it made sense, while some of it did not resonate with me. I do know there are some foods I cannot be around – for example, gummies – however, I am fine with avocados. I learned what a food plan was, which was life-changing. I had been living like Darth Vader, only seeing two sides of life: the Dark Side (bingeing), or being good and restricting, AKA the Light Side (hanging with Luke Skywalker). I had to learn to live.

Twelve-step food programs do amazing work, and their food plans have been of great help to me in terms of developing my own food plan, which you will learn about. Keep in mind, I had gone to Weight Watchers for years, and the meetings are very different, as is the perspective on food. I am telling you about my quest to figure this weight thing the hell out for once and for all. I was so tired of it all.

I read everything I could, became a nutrition nerd, listened to podcasts on the way to after-school pickup, experimented on myself, and came up with a food plan that I find rewarding, nutritionally sound, and that makes me as sane as someone with my personality can be.

Following my quest, my years of starving and dieting and eating in the dark, I finally came across the right combination of foods that fixed my food drama. I want to share it with you, because I do not want anyone else to struggle and I do not want others to have to have the constant food noise in their brain on repeat. I know how important it is to feel living without being on a diet or being out of control is an option. We can live eating food – not obsessing about it, dreaming about it, bingeing on it, or feeling it is out to get us. It is possible for food to be viewed as fuel for our bodies, not a moral issue.

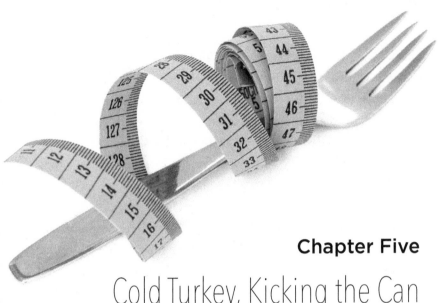

Chapter Five

Cold Turkey, Kicking the Can Down the Road, and Winston Churchill

WINSTON CHURCHILL ONCE SAID "If you're going through hell, keep going." This sums up why I feel going cold turkey when it comes to sugar is the best way to go. Now, before you go running for your secret stashes, hear me out!

We all agree sugar creates a need for more sugar, right? So, if you were to clean up your act for good, the day after the Super Bowl would be good, right? You need to make it an ideal time – after the holidays, so you wouldn't be tempted. Let's say you decided this in the middle of October, but at this point all the pre-holiday food is out. In America, Halloween is a giant candy holiday that usually morphs into

Thanksgiving in late November, then all of December becomes a food fest with Christmas, and New Year's is all about alcohol, and January becomes football, i.e. bar food and alcohol. So by the time of the Super Bowl, which is the first weekend in February, you would have been on a food bender 93 days long, knowing the clock was running down and I was going to take away all of your favorite foods from you any day now. Much like those with the "Last Supper" mentality, it is 93 days for you to cram more sugar into your system. The constant excuses, justifications, and delays are another way of kicking the can down the road. You didn't really want to do something, so you found a million reasons not to. When I really want to do something, I find a way, I know you will be the same way, now that you have decided this is the last time with sugar.

Things change dramatically the first week off of sugar, but your brain and body are still attempting to detox for months, so in the spirit of giving you the best chance to get the most recovery the most quickly, let's not make things worse by going on a "Last Supper" leading up to breaking up with sugar.

Phases of Change

You know that really annoying thing well-meaning people tell you when life has really kicked you in the teeth, that "The only constant is change"? It is true, but for our purposes, there is some science about making changes that you need to know to kick sugar to the curb for good. The same concepts can be used for checking your cellphone too often or buying too many pairs of shoes online when you can't sleep. Change comes in seven phases.

Precontemplation. You are not aware that there is a problem behavior that needs to be changed. In this phase, you are not even connecting the dots between what you are eating and how you are feeling. Eventually, you do, which leads us to **Contemplation.** Maybe you are acknowledging that there is a problem but are not yet ready or sure of wanting to make a change. Perhaps you have read articles on the dangers of sugar in *Self* magazine at the gym, or bought an app to keep track of your sugar consumption. However, you haven't really admitted to yourself you need to break up with sugar, and not get back together, in the immortal words of Taylor Swift, "like ever." Not just until the reunion or until you can fit into your white jeans. You haven't admitted that you and sugar need to see other people. It is not you, it is sugar, and it isn't a matter of timing or whatever clichés we have used to dump people in the past.

When we decide that this is *the* time, no more half-hearted attempts, we move into **Preparation/Determination** (Getting ready to change). This is what we need to do when we decide this isn't just a see-other-people breakup, but a return-all-the-stuff, delete-their-number-out-of-your-phone breakup. You will learn how to take **Action** and to exhibit **Willpower** (Changing behavior) in Chapter Six.

From all of my years of dieting and weight watching, I remember how great it was to get to Maintenance, but the term will mean something different in this book. **Maintenance** (Maintaining the behavior change) is in Chapter Eight. Now I went back and forth with talking about this next chapter because I didn't want you to think that slipping is inevitable and OK. However, it would not be fair to *not* give you skills in preventing **Slip** (Returning to older behaviors and abandoning the new changes), so those are in Chapter 10.

It Is All About Me

I was the type of sugar person who could eat an entire bag of dried mangos on the drive home from Costco. Granted, I worked out a lot, but stopping such behavior has improved my overall health, my mental health, my skin, even my sleep. So, imagine if I was still eating bags of dried mangos and was given warnings by my doctor that something had to stop.

When I was starting to write this book, I had to do a lot of pre-writing exercises. At first, I thought they were unnecessary, but I began to come around and realize my attitude was unhelpful and I went all in on whatever the writing staff told me to do. I started to connect the dots between my clients who would attempt to tell me how it wasn't a big deal if they only ate sugar, flour, and sweetener on their birthday and how I'd resisted the writing exercises. They were finding their own workaround. When a client does this, she is picking and choosing the parts of the plan she feels comfortable with, but she is not fully committing to the food plan.

The reason we do this is because if we do not fully commit, we still reserve the right to have a little bit of independence. If we do not succeed, it was because we weren't fully trying anyway. So, no biggie right? When we are all in, we do whatever the expert tells us to do. Why? Because they know what they are talking about and it might not make sense at the time to us, but all will be revealed eventually. I observed my resistance to the exercises was because I thought I knew everything about my reader, so why do I have to do all the silly exercises? It was not because I did not care about her (my ideal reader) it was because she and I were already BFFs who threw slumber parties and braided each other's hair. This is the same side of the coin as when clients tell me they are going to go "off" their plan on their birthdays, but not to worry because they will be "good" when they get back.

So to circle back to my writing exercises, once I got over myself, if the writing staff had told me to set up a stand at Grand Central Station during rush hour like Lucy from *Peanuts* that said "Ask me how to lose weight," I would have. I needed to be committed to that level. I didn't need to have a back-up plan of how I could still retain my imagined coolness because being committed to self-improvement is the coolest thing we can do for ourselves. What gives us greater independence than loving ourselves?

One of the things I had to do was to figure out who I was writing this book for. I couldn't be writing a book for everyone. You can't be everything for everyone, and quite frankly, it is impossible. I have no idea what it is like to be morbidly obese and unable to leave my house. I could still empathize with them as a person in pain, put them on a food plan, and find one of my much better equipped colleagues to come in and take it from there.

My training is as a holistic health coach and a food addiction counselor. I will break them down so you have a little more understanding as to how they are different and how they apply to why I want you to white knuckle this.

Health coaches are taught to look at life *holistically*. For example, you could be eating the freshest, most organic food in the world, but if you are in a toxic relationship with your romantic partner and you are constantly stressed out, fighting, breaking up, and getting back together – how healthy can you truly be? All parts of your life are impacted by the others. To circle back to our dilemma with our diet, the sooner you get your weight under control, the quicker the rest of your life will come into balance. Imagine how much more time you will have without the constant diet noise in your brain monopolizing your attention? The additional space can be used for things like reading for pleasure, or remembering where you put your keys, or journaling. Something other than managing the latest high glycemic carbohydrate influx and subsequent and inevitable crash. Keeping one step ahead of the food is time-consuming.

My education as a food addiction counselor is focused on full-blown *food addiction*. As of today, food addiction isn't seen as a true medical diagnosis by the medical community. It is seen as a process addiction, the same as compulsive gambling, even though it is a chemical in the same way alcohol or heroin is. I am not going to bother to tell you the politics behind this or why I believe the situation to be the way it is. In recent years, food addiction clinics have been popping up and traditional addiction clinics have added food dependency as one of their offerings. The numbers of people who self-identify as food addicts are staggering. Science has known it for a long time, and I am predicting the mainstream will soon acknowledge how food truly impacts our brains and how addicting it can be.

What is important for you today is to know that food addiction isn't just a concept thrown around in twelve-step food recovery programs or on binge-eating podcasts. It has a place in discussing sugar. The important part about food addiction and how it matters to us is that food addicts are at the end of the spectrum of eating disorders because they are chemically addicted to the substances in certain foods. These addictive substances are in things such as sugar, flour, and processed food. The takeaway for those of us who have struggled with sugar is to know that sugar chemically has had a hold on us and it is not made up, or a matter of willpower, or of being a good person.

Sugar is eight times more addictive than cocaine, to go back to our rats from Chapter Four. Food addicts are genetically and environmentally more susceptible than others to becoming addicted to these chemicals. There are many, many theories as to what came first with addiction; basically, it is like the old chicken-and-the-egg debate. Again, that is not the focus of this book. This is your book on how to break up with sugar for good. The way to solve sugar today is to rip the Band-Aid off in one swift move, white knuckle it, ghost it – pick your favorite metaphor because we are going to detox already!!!

Darth Vader and Me

I was tired of seeing the world in black or white. I was either being good – i.e. dieting or starving myself – or being bad and doing laps in a sugar lake. I was not just living. I began to relate to Darth Vader, which is super weird. I have seen *Star Wars* and the various prequels and sequels way too many times, but there is some symmetry to his story that I did find a little connection with.

Anakin was born a good kid, life happened, he got angry, hung out with the wrong crowd, became Darth Vader, Natalie Portman dumped him, then he went bad for a very long time. He turned it around right before the end, after his son talked some sense into him. He was never just a life in the middle you know, like Han Solo. Let's be honest here: Han Solo isn't super good, or super bad. He's charming and all that, but he's somewhere in the middle. That is a food plan. We will go over food plans in Chapter Seven in greater detail. Food plans are your Han Solo, a devilishly handsome way to get through life. Never boring, but not as volatile as life on the dark side or as pure and unattainable as a lifetime of dieting or life as a monk like Luke Skywalker.

The Two Questions

In the TV show *The Walking Dead*, they used to have three questions before they would take on a new member of their good-guys squad. These questions were used to weed out the yahoos and to see if the interviewee (is there such a thing in a post-apocalyptic world?) Was honest.

In sugar, (as a reminder, I am including flour and sweetener) these are the only two questions that matter:

1. Do you believe food has addictive properties?
2. Do you believe you have shown symptoms of having a chemical reaction to food?

After reading to this point, you've seen a great deal of research and my own experiences with sugar being addictive. You might be starting to have the sinking feeling that this book isn't about finding the magic pill for weight loss, but that the first class ticket to ending food drama is eliminating sugar, flour, and sweetener. This is the only way I know to work for myself, my clients, and the friends I have helped.

You might be having an internal dialogue right now where you are making a list of all the people you know who have managed to keep weight off, yet are still the moderation types. You are mostly sure sugar, flour, and sweetener are still in their lives but they are not tortured by it. Remember, appearances can be deceiving. If you were sitting in front of me with your list of magical mythical creatures, I would ask you why you are taking so much time to argue with the idea that sugar, flour, and sweetener are the problem. If moderation works for them, that is great for them – and I am sure, if we sat down together and made a list of all the people we knew who went on a diet, thought they were in the clear, went back to eating "how they wanted," gained it all back and then some, my list would be about ten times longer than yours.

What do you have to lose by giving sugar up for 60 days? The time will pass whether or not you decide this is the last time you eat sugar. Now we know what the other way – eating sugar – is like. The other way is why you picked up the book. The other way is what kept me in the diet cycle for the majority of my adult life. The other way is a quick way to nowhere.

Now imagine we are 60 days from today and you have given up sugar, flour, and sweetener. I know what this scenario looks like as well. You might not be able to envision it, which I completely understand. I couldn't see it, but I knew I wanted it. Let me tell you about it since I am there now. I do not wake up thinking, "Oh crap, what did I eat yesterday." I do not worry if my fall clothes will fit now that summer is really over and I am changing my closets in and out. My skin is clear and my mood is stable. I am much more confident than I was before and I do not live in fear of having to get weighed at the doctor's office if I get a cold.

I understand the reason why we hold on so tightly to the other way. A dear friend of mine Hillary, who I met in Weight Watchers, will every so often say she wants to meet for coffee and this time she is really going to lose the weight, will I help her? I always say yes, we meet, I tell her I still do not think sugar, flour, and sweetener are an option for her. Hillary will listen and tell me she needs to think about it. A few days will pass, and when I call to check in on her for something unrelated, she doesn't pick up. Always texts back.

When we do speak, I never bring up the coffee date we had or how she never got back to me about giving up the problematic foods. Why do I not bring it up? First of all, she is a dear friend. Secondly, she is still in Contemplation. She knows what she is supposed to do but does not want to do it. She wants to have her cake and eat it too. She wants to weigh what she weighed when she got married 20 years ago, but she wants to eat like she does now. I can't give that to her.

Hillary contacted me a week ago and we had the same exact conversation only this time it was on text. She said she was going to go to Weight Watchers in the morning because "They let me keep sugar, and flour." I asked her why that was so important to her and she said because she loves them, she is Italian, and I will take them away. I asked her if she ever thought the reason why she lost some weight and gained it back and then some each and every time with Weight Watchers is because she kept the sugar and flour in the mix? This conversation went back and forth and I told Hillary if she was serious, I would help her but only if she was all in. She needed to listen to what I recommended and not have any of the moderation ideas in her head. I told her to call me the next day if she was serious. What do you think happened? I am sure you know, but just to go on the record, she did not call and Hillary is not picking up the phone. Hillary just told me she recommitted and has lost 6.2 lbs in a month. I told her I was happy for her, meanwhile my latest current group of new clients have lost double that in the same amount of time, but that is OK. She will let me know when she is ready. In the meantime, I will love her just the same.

If you have had headaches, mood swings, and/or acne, mild depression, trouble sleeping, and you can connect the dots to your intake of sugar … you have been impacted by the chemical properties of sugar. I am not saying you are a good or bad person, or that you need to go to a therapist to talk about your feelings about food. I am saying – with complete certainty – that you are presenting reasons to break up with sugar.

I am very aware of my own limitations; for example, I am awful at cardio kickboxing, I cannot puffy paint to save my life, and my pancakes are awful. I am confident in what I do know. I know what it is like to be a thirty-or forty-something woman who cannot get it together due to food. Period. End of Discussion. From the outside, things were great. I had cute kids, I worked professionally, had accomplished a lot, and was a super Mommy. I had a cute husband and plenty of stuff, I even looked the part down to my designer athleisure clothes and my hybrid SUV. However, I was freaking miserable and was stuffing my face with canned leftover frosting when the kids were watching *Toy Story* in the other room. Hmmm… how good can things be?

I was teaching spin and yoga and had a bag of Sour Jelly Bellies in the car and could not wait to get back to them as soon as I finished up the meditation bit on inhaling the good and exhaling the bad or whatever. *Ugh*, why is this woman stopping to talk to me after class? Thankfully, that didn't take long. I wonder if I sounded authentic when I was discussing loving yourself *for yourself?*

The Final Question

When my daughter was around thirteen months, she knew a grand total of three words. They were "up," "hi," and "uh-oh." She and I went on a cross-country plane trip and she was a very unhappy flyer and she repeated "UPUPUPUPUPUPUPUPUPUPUPUPUP" pretty much until she passed out from exhaustion about two hours into the six-hour plane ride. I got her point: She wanted the heck out of her restraining device, she was not enjoying flying the friendly skies, and quite frankly, she was over it.

In the words of Barack Obama, "We are the change that we seek." It isn't as if you had no idea sugar wasn't healthy for you before you picked up this book. Now, I want to know your reason for wanting to change now – what is your Why – and, more importantly, I want you to write it down. Why is your Why important now? What is your reason for wanting to break up with sugar now? Why *why why why why why why why why why why*? Do you get my point? Your Why really matters. It matters more than getting out of that car seat did to my toddler. It is so crucial because you will need to check in with it on a regular basis. It must be self-focused. Maybe the title of my book caught your eye or you heard good things and you decided the time was right to finally give it up. If the reason is for anything other than yourself, it will not last. If your reason for wanting to make a lasting change has to do with pleasing your boyfriend or because you heard a celebrity does not eat sugar, it will not take. The reason needs to be about you or it will not work. To use an over-used saying, the only thing you can control is yourself, so why do you want this? What is your Why? Write down your Why. If your mind is a blank, or there are too many whys to find one, maybe telling you mine will help.

I was so stinking tired of the sugar drama. I was exhausted from the emotional roller coaster of always waking up hating myself, of finding candy wrappers in my secret spots, of trying to get through the day not eating sugar only to give in by around 2 p.m. or die (or want to) of a pounding headache. I was over-eating one way in public and another by myself. My daughter was getting older and I didn't want her to realize mom was full of it when it came to what I told her to eat versus what I really did consume. I didn't care if I lost weight, or if my skin cleared up, or if I never had six-pack abs, I just wanted the sugar drama to end in my brain. The mental crap had to leave. So my Why would have been: to find peace.

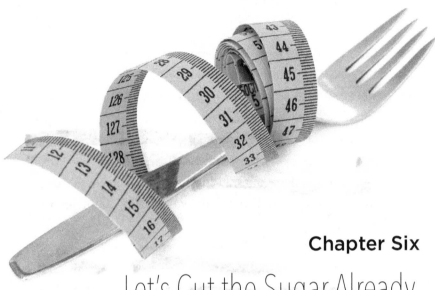

Chapter Six

Let's Cut the Sugar Already, AKA Take Some Action

SO TO RECAP, we know why sugar isn't working for us, we know what sugar has done to us, and we know why we want to break up with sugar – now we just need to break up with it already.

Find your why, then use it to channel your Motivation.
- Jerrod Morris

So, how do we do it?

1. Write down your main Why. You will know this backwards and forwards. Sort of like your Social Security Number in college. I am not saying you want to share it with everyone you know,

but I want it to be in the forefront of your brain at least 3-5 times a day. I want you to connect with it before each meal, when you wake up, and when you go to sleep. What will make you not eat the cookie when no one else is looking? For me, it was rationally knowing what the sugar would chemically do to me, and emotionally knowing how disappointed I would be with myself if I went backwards. It was that simple. It can be that simple for you. Feel free to take my Why until you have your own.

2. Write down any other Whys you are giving up sugar. They can be as simple as "to feel better in my clothes," or "I want to be as healthy as I can be for my kids." Remember your main Why needs to be about you.

3. Make the conscious decision food is not worth your peace of mind, your health, or any other top reasons. I always tell my spin students "choose your choice." Now many of them would tell you that I am the hardest teacher on the face of the planet, but that I always give them results, I never have them do anything I have not done before, and I know their names, their life stories, and who loves Dave Matthews Band. For the last three years, I have taught an early morning Friday class. In the Northeast, it can be pretty stinking dark at 6:15 a.m., and you have to really want it to get up and drive in the dark to come and see me in January. These participants of mine "chose their choice" – they didn't just flirt with getting into the NYC marathon, or losing the weight, or finally being the fastest person in their age bracket on their biking team (all results I have gotten them), they committed. I have to bring my A game for them – they deserve it and they bring theirs to me. They are all in, and so am I, or else our Friday a.m. relationship would not work. We

all had to make the decision – the conscious choice – so make yours.

4. Throw away everything in your house, car, at work, your secret stashes, and anything tempting. I know that there are foods a normal person wouldn't find to be a problem, but I have been known to overeat in a pinch. I cannot have golden raisins, Lucky Charms, or Pirate's Booty in my pantry. Now, all of that stuff needs to go. If you live alone, congrats!! If you are like most of us, who have roommates or live with family members or partners, you have to figure something out. Find alternatives that you do not like and get them for your family members. I have found there are pretty much two ways people deal with this one. I have had clients who have found it difficult to control themselves around pizza, so they chose to not be in situations involving pizza as much as possible. Then their romantic partner would order pizza in front of them and say something to the effect of "Well, I do not have a problem with it, so why can't I have pizza?" Your partner is more than welcome to have pizza they can do it at work, at a bar with friends, or anywhere on earth where you aren't for the time being. As far as we know the world isn't ending and pizza isn't going anywhere.

5. Be aware we do not live in a vacuum; however, we can reasonably control our environment as much as possible. Back to my client and the pizza and the partner. Be reasonable. If you go somewhere that has pizza, such as a pizza party with five-year-olds, you cannot get too testy with the host for having pizza there. However, if you are ordering at a fancy restaurant, feel free to ask the waiter if the salad dressing has any sugar in it. If they do not know, have them find out. You are paying the bill and you are breaking up with sugar for good, after all.

6. Get support ahead of time. Tell a few trusted people that are supportive, that get it, and that you can easily reach if you are having a bad day. I do not encourage making a public proclamation – what is the rush? You can always run an ad in Sunday's NY Times in a few months. The paper will gladly take your advertisement dollars next quarter.

7. Look at your calendar for the next three weeks. Anything major coming up? Travel, holiday stress, in-laws visiting? Start to think of what food related issues – such as the candy around Easter – will add to the pressure of your in-laws visiting. Give some attention to what you can do ahead of time to make things less pressure-filled. Could you invite your in-laws to stay in a nearby hotel? How about you tell your kids the Easter Bunny is just delivering toys this year? Maybe you let your friend host the neighborhood egg decorating party. My point is, plan ahead and be willing to get creative.

Now What?

One of the many questions I get as a food coach/counselor/exercise teacher is "So what do you eat?" It is especially entertaining when a client runs into me where they think I am not supposed to be. You know, such as at a party or a bar. Many times, they will act like a drunk sorority girl and give me a giant hug, tell me they love me, and attempt to distract me from noticing what they were consuming by asking me why I am not at the gym. They must think of me the way I thought of my first-grade teacher when I ran into her at the grocery store, as only existing in one part of their life.

What I do eat is pretty simple. It isn't anything fancy or things you cannot get at a normal grocery store in a normal town in a normal part of North America. So, don't worry that I am going to be sending you to super-expensive health food stores to buy extravagant or strange ingredients. This is important to me for a couple of reasons. First of all, I grew up in a town in Central California with 10,000 people. Dogs would sleep in the street. Seriously, they would sleep in the street and everyone would drive around them. We didn't have a Starbucks until after I left for college. However, we had a farmers' market and we had traditional grocery stores. A life free from food drama is not just for those who live in trendy urban neighborhoods.

Secondly, my food plan isn't only for the people who can afford and can be bothered to locate an ostrich egg to make a special omelet, as preached by a certain blond celebrity. The food plan is for everyone, including those of us who could not find an ostrich egg if we had to, and those of us who would not, on principle.

Lastly, the food plan is practical. If all of a sudden, I have to go to my mother's, I do not want to have to ship special food or try to get the right salad dressing thorough TSA. I want to be able to go to a regular Albertson's, Fred Meyer, Dominick's, Stop N Shop, or Kroger, depending on where in the USA I am. In all of these various grocery store chains, I can find broccoli, full-fat dairy, organic milk, and chicken. It might not be the exact kind I would get at home in the New York City area, but I will be fine.

I eat a lot of protein and fat, and little carbs. I eat three hearty meals a day, and do not eat past dinner, which I try to keep around 7 p.m. This got me and keeps me off of sugar and it will for you as well. I do not drink diet soda, diet drinks or anything with the word diet in it. I do not use fake sweetener, artificial flavorings, or fake butter.

When you first break up with sugar, it is important you follow these four guidelines. This works for me and it works for my clients. I have tested this exact food plan on women our age, with our food issues, and this has worked miracles. Not my word, theirs.

My Four Guidelines to a Clean Breakup

We have all witnessed a messy breakup. Maybe you have been a part of one. I was in one that took way too long in college, but that is so another story for another day. This breakup needs to be swift and clean. You and sugar are done. There is none of the ending-as-friends talk. Your mindset is very important. So, your mind needs to be made up: This is it. I believe you can do it.

The purpose of this food plan (note I didn't write diet) is to get you off of all processed food, wheat, grain, and added sugar. A meal or a food plan is how we live life, not something we go on and off like a merry-go-round. This road map will keep you satisfied and full.

One: Three Meals a Day

Breakfast, Lunch, and Dinner

I do not want you snacking all day. You will survive between dinner and breakfast, I guarantee it. When you are eating enough fat and protein, you will not be starving between meals. Lots of sugar in processed food will make you feel hungry, due to the blood-sugar swings. This will not happen post breakup. I didn't believe it was possible. I was one of those people that always rolled my eyes when people would tell me they didn't get hungry between meals, since I couldn't go from breakfast to lunch ever, especially if I worked out. Of course, I usually chose something awful – like a latte full of artificial sweeteners – and then I would add a few sweetener packets. Since coffee didn't really count, I usually had some sort of sugar-infused healthy bar in my purse or there was always the candy in the car. Between meals, I do not want you to be having anything other than tea, black coffee, or water.

My macronutrient goals each day are 40 percent fat, 40 percent protein, 20 percent carbohydrates. This keeps me full and satisfied. I am able to go from dinner at 7 p.m. until breakfast at 8 a.m., no problem. That was impossible when I was eating low fat/high carb. If you want to, download one of the apps that will count your macros. I like MyFitnessPal and no, they don't give me a cut of the profits.

Do not starve yourself in the morning and eat a giant dinner. I am not a big calorie counter, but I just looked at my last week's stats and my three meals were not that different in caloric weight. Oh, and we are on vacation as I write this. Vacation is a loose term, as any woman who has rented a house with four children at the beach will tell you.

Your last meal is three hours before bed, if not more. After that last meal of the night, your eating is done for the day. The kitchen is closed. You can have decaffeinated tea or water. If you have an urge to eat, you are bored, or restless, or need to call a girlfriend, or go watch *The Hot Housewives of Rancho Cucamonga*. Whatever it is, it isn't physical – there is no way you'll be hungry with the amount of high quality food you will be eating.

I used to have this weird sensation that until something sweet came into my mouth, the food day wasn't over, so I would have no choice but to look around for something to satisfy that need, or so I told myself. That went away when I started following the Four Guidelines. I have little habits or rituals now to distract myself when my old habits are calling my name. In my house, the bedrooms are on the second floor, so after dinner, I go upstairs for the rest of the night. I drink a giant mug of tea, then I will brush and floss my teeth, then put in my TMJ retainer. It isn't cute, but it has stopped all the mindless eating.

Two: Plan Your Meals Ahead

I will decide the night before what I am eating for the day.

There are a couple of reasons why I do this: If I try and wing it, bad things can happen. For example, I get too hungry when I hit the grocery store and make awful choices. Another possibility is I am too overwhelmed, cannot even deal with the grocery store, and I eat whatever I can find at home, which isn't usually a balanced meal and is typically eaten standing with the fridge open.

Planning ahead makes you aware of any possible obstacles before you get there. If I decide I am having fish tacos tomorrow night for dinner, and check in the fridge and realize the fish is frozen tonight, I have enough time to defrost it. If I chose to shoot from the hip, I would have nothing but a giant fish popsicle tomorrow at dinner time and who knows what my bad habit brain would have told me was a good idea to eat.

If I am going out, I can check the menu ahead of time. I also do this for clients. I had one just yesterday go to a Mets game and I looked up Citi Field and figured out five different things she could eat on her food plan other than a hot dog with fake cheese and cookie dough. I found out there is a fruit stand at the baseball stadium. Planning ahead gives you a chance to prepare like this.

It is also more cost- and time-efficient to realize you can use the chicken breasts in tomorrow's fajitas and the drumsticks for the kids' lunch than to keep running to the grocery store. When we are calmer, we make better choices, and our body is able to absorb the nutrients better. It is a win-win all around.

Each night, I write down my actual food. Here's what I ate on 8/24/2017:

B-Avocado, tomatoes with bacon, and a side of fruit

L-Leftover steak, 1/2 sweet potato, pat of butter, hummus, cucumber, and tomatoes

D- Crab cakes, large green salad, dressing, steamed spinach with olive oil

Three: Whole, Real Food

To keep it simple, stick to the perimeter of your grocery store. So you will be eating fruits and vegetables, legumes, animal proteins, and dairy products (if you tolerate them).

Do not consume anything made in a lab, or synthetic fake foods, AKA frozen diet meals, funky nutrition bars with 45 ingredients, or diet or fat-free dairy. I want you to eat real food because your body knows what to do with it. Our bodies know how to digest an apple. Something made in a lab to fake our brains into thinking it is sweet but isn't will cause a reaction of some sort to the rest of our bodies, and most of the time the reaction is not cute or pleasant. Oh, and our brain is still looking for that apple.

Diet Coke has a special place in my heart because it was a mainstay in my college years. My sorority sisters and I would go to the local 7-11 (or, as we called it, "Sevies") and for $.69 get a 72-ounce Diet Coke from a fountain machine. I did this all the time. I had no idea the soda was the reason why I was always hungry, a tad chubby, and would eat bags of gummy bears. Never mind all the damage diet soda does to your body, your teeth, and just about every other part of your body. Stay away from diet soda, fake sweetener, and all such chemicals.

For a list of the grocery store staples I recommend keeping on hand year-round, go to my Appendix.

Four: Protein, Fiber, Fat, and Low-Glycemic Carbs, Each and Every Time You Eat

This will likely be easy for you to remember: You have four main guidelines for eating, and four boxes to check each and every time you have a meal.

Each meal needs to have:

- Protein *Cottage cheese, chicken, lean beef*
- Fiber *fruit, veg (not potatoes, corn, carrots)*
- Fat *butter, oil*
- A low-glycemic carb, *L carb bread*

Protein: I want you to get the best quality protein you can find and afford. Fish, eggs, chicken, beef, soy, nuts, seeds, eggs, low-fat or regular-fat dairy. I have friends who make the time and have the desire to go to farmers' markets and talk to the local farmers and really get to know where all of their food comes from, which is fabulous. My family orders meat from an organic farmer, and it comes in a giant frozen block once a month, and it goes into the freezer, to be defrosted accordingly. It is on automatic payment now, which is good, as I tend to be over-scheduled. I pay attention to the most polluted fish lists, but it took me years to remember which type of salmon is the bad one. I eat locally as often as possible, so when I am in Maryland, I eat blue crab. When I am in Maine, I eat lobster. Try to eat animal protein with the least amount of miles as possible.

If you are a vegetarian or a vegan, there is no reason you cannot stick to the food plan. Just be sure to get enough protein in the form of nuts, seeds, beans, and/or soy. Yes, you read that correctly, soy. Now, studies have shown soy can be problematic. Sure, if used in junk food such as soy ice cream, and you have been advised by a doctor to not eat soy, then find another source of protein. I tend to eat some type of animal protein at almost every meal. I have gone through phases where I did not eat animal protein for a variety of reasons, and have ended up returning to a meal plan with animal protein.

Fiber: back in the day we used to think of fiber as bran. Actually, fiber is in most vegetables and fruit. Every time you eat, I want you to make sure you have some sort of fiber in your meals. That could mean throwing avocado into a smoothie or having a side of broccoli with dinner.

Fat: You will be eating real butter, real cream, and fully leaded salad dressing. Do not be afraid of fat. If you are hungry before dinner, 99 percent of the time it was because you did not have enough fat at lunch. If you are famished at 4:00 p.m., I will have my clients have some fat, such as decaf coffee with cream, 1/2 an avocado, or even a chicken drumstick with skin under the understanding that this is a one-time thing and we will discuss what they could have done.

Carbs: Yep, I did write carbs. Low-glycemic carbohydrates as in sweet potatoes, berries, spaghetti squash, pretty much all vegetables and fruit. The lower on the glycemic index, the better. As a reminder, the glycemic scale measures carbohydrates according to how they affect blood glucose levels. Not all carbohydrates are created equal. For example, a baked potato measures 111 and a yam is 54 on the glycemic scale. Both are starches, but the baked potato will spike your blood sugar twice as fast as a yam. There is a link in the Appendix as well.

Keys to the Kingdom

I have found eating a high fat, low carbohydrate meal plan keeps me satisfied between meals, away from sugar and able to maintain my weight without giving it tons of extra thought or effort. I remember my days of serious dieting where I felt like I was holding back the tide when it came to maintaining a weight loss, the way I eat now it doesn't require such mental work. I am not counting down the minutes until I can eat next, as I can always find protein, fat and a low glycemic carbohydrate in any restaurant or buffet. Eating this way has made my life easier on so many levels, and it will for you as well. When I developed my food plan, it wasn't from any one source, but many and I believe it to the best out there. It is simple, straightforward, economical and easy to remember.

I came to these guidelines through lots of formal education, many twelve-step meetings, a lot of trial and error on myself, listening to clients, and patience. I am giving you the keys to my kingdom, so to speak. From my training as a health coach, I realized I needed to address the emotional part of sugar. Just fixing the symptom isn't solving the problem. As a food addiction counselor, I became aware of the brain and how sugar hijacks it, which is why I came up with a zero tolerance policy with it. The twelve-step meetings taught me how to live life not on a diet or on a binge, the concept of a food plan was introduced to me. My years of dieting, having sugar hangovers and Monday-morning diets have given me great insight as to what didn't work, no matter how hard I tried or attempted to force a solution. Lastly, my clients helped me a great deal. I had many versions of my food plan, I kept testing it and testing it until it got everyone off of sugar for good. It reminded me of Goldilocks and eventually we found the right combination of food, structure, and planning that was just right.

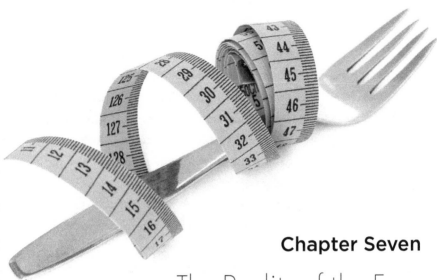

Chapter Seven

The Reality of the Four Guidelines and Four Checkboxes

SO WE HAVE GONE OVER how we got here, how we dumped sugar for good, how we are going to stay broken up and our Why. However, for the process of breaking up, let's drill down a little more into what your life will look like as a single woman, free and clear of sugar.

One: Three Meals a Day

Breakfast, Lunch, and Dinner

Now, I know many of us have heard recommendations to eat every couple of hours, or to have mini-meals, or that a certain food addiction clinic has their people eat a large snack as a metabolic boost before bed. Remember the food trends of ten years ago? The Master Cleanse (lemon, maple syrup, and cayenne pepper) was big to lose tons of weight in a short period of time, which of course meant it came back with a vengeance. Do hundred-calorie snack packs ring a bell? They were little bags of a hundred calories of processed something. I can show you the escalating obesity rates, along with the increased amounts of processed sugar in America, if you still think these are a good idea. My point in this walk down memory lane of food trends past is this mini-meal and eating-all-day theory is a fad. To eat all day is not necessary – it is taxing on your body to constantly be processing food, and to go to sleep on a full stomach is bad for digestion.

Think of our grandparents: They ate three meals a day – and you know what, they were thinner, generally healthier, and ate higher quality food, even without the miracle of the Internet. Three meals a day is sufficient to sustain you if they have enough fat and protein. Back in my low fat/high carb weight watching days, I could barely make it to 10:00 a.m. when I had some sort of low fat/high carb snack because I was starving. Now, I have a high fat/low carb breakfast and I am fine until lunch; sometimes, I could honestly go a little longer than lunchtime but I don't, because I do not want to be bothered to stop and eat later. Seriously, I have become one of those alien people who have to remember to stop and eat? I never understood those people, I always thought they were faking it or, quite frankly, something was wrong with them. Perhaps they naturally ate the way it took me decades to come to – or they came from Mars.

Now, when you are eating three meals a day, there are some things to be aware of. First of all, your body will adapt long before your mind will. You have years of habits of snacking to get rid of. I like to imagine a giant carpet where you have walked a certain way for 20 or so years. To go from door A to door B you always walked a certain path. Now you are going to walk a different path, and it will take a while for your brain to catch up with your feet. There will be days where right around your normal snack time you might find yourself bored or just sort of looking for that break in the day that a snack would fix. Well, that is change happening! Go get a giant glass of water and check in with your Why. Remember the numerous reasons you decided this time was the last time.

If you occasionally have brunch, no big deal. However, the majority of the time, have three meals, spaced apart, with at least three hours between lunch and dinner and between dinner and bed. After dinner, you are done. Even on Christmas or your birthday or on days that end in Y. Excuses and exceptions are a slippery slope, so do not even go there.

Two: Meal Planning

I will decide the night before what I am eating for the day, or if I am super-organized (which happens, you know, as often as an eclipse), the week.

The main reason I do this:

The annoying yet wise saying "When we fail to plan, we plan to fail," is so accurate with me, I cannot even tell you. When I would go to the grocery store right after a spin class, nothing good would come of it. I was working my first job and I went to the 5:30 p.m. class every night and then would go to the grocery store and make really bad choices every single day. Not only was I way too hungry – and by this point, wearing gross clothing and wanting to get the heck out of the grocery store – the frenetic energy of a grocery store at 7 p.m. on a workday is usually pretty chaotic, and does not lead to great healthy choices. I did not have a list or a plan, I was just grazing. I have memories of gnawing on a Powerbar in my car, then eating sourdough and hummus for dinner, and eating Ben &Jerry's Phish Food at night. I cringe when I think of those days, but they are a good teaching tool for my clients. I have a seasonal grocery list on my smartphone, so I do not act like the Tasmanian Devil on Pop Rocks when I walk into the store.

If I plan what I am going to eat the night before, it is less likely anything crazy will happen. Worst-case scenario, I realize I need to make a run to the store that night for the morning, but it is not as if I need the ingredient immediately. The sense of urgency and drama has been dramatically reduced. I also have more time to research recipes and not get into ruts which can lead to boredom and unhappiness with my food plan.

Three: Whole, Real Food

There is a scene in *Back to the Future 2*, where Marty, played by Michael J. Fox, goes to the future of 2015, and the food is similar to what he was eating in 1985, but due to the modern innovations, it is better. Pizza was dehydrated, and then through magic, AKA a re-hydrator, it is full-sized. Clearly, that innovation didn't happen along with the flying cars, but it does illustrate how the current food isn't necessarily better than the food that once was.

I am a big fan of sticking to the rails or the perimeter of the grocery store. Most grocery stores are laid out the same: You walk into the produce section, the meat is on the back wall, and dairy is parallel to the produce. Now everything in the middle is typically processed food. In there you have Wheat Thins, Ding Dongs, vanilla wafers, fish sticks, Funfetti cake mixes, and things featuring words like "cheez."

There are many problems with processed foods: They are usually full of high-fructose corn syrup and various types of sugar, they are hyper-rewarding which leads to over-eating, they contain artificial and/or controversial ingredients, they are more likely to be addictive than real foods, processed foods are usually another term for sugar, they rarely have any nutrients or fiber, our bodies convert them to body fat easier than real food, and they are often full of trans-fat, clogging our arteries.

Four: Protein, Fiber, Fat, and Low-Glycemic Carbs, Each and Every Time You Eat

Now when I first heard about low carbs back in the early 2000s, it was in the heyday of Atkins. I remember my friend's husband eating hot dogs dipped in mayonnaise before their wedding to lose weight. Of course, the weight found him after the honeymoon and brought many friends to stay. The balanced meal and four food groups paradigm we grew up with has way more to do with USDA politics and subsidies than science and nutrition, so I am not going to bother going into it. What I want to discuss with you is science and nutrition. To have a meal with protein, fiber, fat, and a low-glycemic carb will keep your blood stream balanced, you will stay full, you will have a happy GI tract, you will lose weight if you need to, chronic inflammation will decrease if not completely go away, any weight you lose is more likely to be from your abdomen which is considered dangerous, and you will break up with sugar for good.

I want to take time to discuss low-glycemic carbohydrates with you. This is not a permission slip to go crazy with the bread bowl. Examples of low-glycemic carbohydrates are sweet potatoes, spaghetti squash, berries, grapefruits, beans, and oats. Most vegetables are low-glycemic; the exceptions are potatoes and corn. The problem with potatoes and corn is that they can be processed by our bodies as sugar, so view them as such and stay away. Back to low-glycemic carbohydrates – a small amount at each meal is key to your blood sugar control and your sanity, and they have fiber. Fiber fills you up, keeps things moving in your GI tract, lowers your cholesterol, and helps control our blood sugar.

Back in my Weigh Watcher days, fiber was having a moment. The idea was the more fiber in something, the less calories, so bring it on! However, scientists can add all the fiber they want into a chocolate cake, it will not eliminate the huge amounts of sugar, fat, and flour from being absorbed. The fiber might slow it down, but it cannot magically turn the cake into a healthy food. You are not looking for fiber added to unhealthy foods; what you want is whole, real foods that naturally contain fiber. For example, broccoli and avocados naturally have fiber without any interference from scientists in a lab. There is no manipulation to trick our body into having us feel full or lowering cholesterol, the whole foods naturally start the process during digestion.

Why Can't I Do It My Way?

I have seen at around day 30 or so, many of my clients start to have a mental rebellion against me and the structure of this program. They start to rebel first in their head (remember where our thoughts go, our everything else follows) and then come the questions and challenges. "Why can't I make a fake cookie out of applesauce and oats?" or "Why won't you let me have a cheat day like this other plan?" Which reminds me of my kids asking, "Why are you so mean?" The reason I am thwacking these ideas down with a giant padded hammer ala whack-a-mole is where these deals and workarounds got you in the past: right into a ditch.

So before you ask, here are my reasons for why the answer is *No* and will always be *No*. Look at your #1 if you need another reason, and if you are not convinced, find #2.

Why Can't I Do It Fat-Free?

Back in the early 90s, American consumers were told eating fat meant you would become, and I hate to use this term, you know, the dreaded three-letter f-word... *fat*. All foods were then touted for being fat-free, foods such as Gummy Bears and bagels were now "good" because they had little to no fat, never mind the glycemic load or the sugar content. Fat was considered the problem, and many of us, including yours truly, got a tad chubby during this phase.

Fat serves a few different purposes in food. It is naturally occurring in animal protein. For example, a skinless, boneless, roasted chicken breast is dry due to the lack of fat in the meat. Removing all fat from a baked good can have a negative impact on how well the dry ingredients bind together. In a brownie, to replace all the fat with nonfat Greek yogurt will create a chocolate goo that cannot hold its shape like a traditional brownie. Yes, it is fat-free, but it is no longer a brownie. I am not sure what we could call it, but a brownie wouldn't be an accurate term.

In recent years, we have learned that sugar and processed foods are a greater cause of concern in the modern diet than the f-word, *fat*, ever was. Sugar and processed foods are reported for causing the obesity, heart disease, and cancer epidemics. In every developing country, once these types of foods are introduced, in a few years the increase of obesity and diabetes goes from anecdotal to substantial; it takes a little longer for heart disease to arrive and then, finally, cancer.

What about Cheat Days?

No to cheat days! If you have successfully weaned yourself off of sugar, why on earth would you start again? Remember, sugar creates the need for more sugar. If you were to have 45 days or so sugar-free, then decide a hot fudge sundae was a great idea, a lot of things would be going on in your body and brain, pre, during, and post the food. You would be more likely to have that hot fudge sundae turn into a full-fledged sugar episode and be more likely to continue, given how happy your body would be with the reintroduction of our frenemy. It would taste better than we remember due to the euphoric recall and how our taste buds have had a chance to recover. None of which would be conducive to breaking up with sugar for good. It comes down to would I rather have the giant cupcake or be sane? For me, sanity from the food drama is worth it, and it will always be. For years, I didn't make peace my choice – and that is why nothing ever took for long.

Reintroduce the White Stuff?

Why can't we reintroduce gummy bears? It is because if you want to stick to your food plan and keep the food drama away, for you, the myth of moderation is playing with fire. First of all, the concept of reintroduction comes from those who have food allergies or intolerances. For example, if someone is having extreme eczema flare-ups, they might go on a FODMAP diet which is very strict anti-inflammatory, even eliminating tomatoes and eggplants. After 30 or 60 days, a food is slowly reintroduced and then everyone waits a week to see if the eczema comes back.

Reintroducing junky processed food because we used to like eating it, is not the same thing as the anti-inflammatory person with the skin issues. Two very different concepts. Reintroducing sugar is a close cousin to idea of going back to eating how we want after the diet is over – it does not work. File it under the old way of thinking, living, and eating.

Or Faux Cookies?

This I get all the time. Usually it involves a recipe they ran across where they can replace chocolate chips with cocoa powder and applesauce instead of sugar, and it goes on and on. This is the deal, why go there? Haven't you had enough cookies in your life to know what they taste like? What they feel like when you digest them? What is your body and brain telling you 15 minutes later? Why would you want to make a fake one, which would only trick your body into thinking this sort of food is still an option, and maybe one day instead of the weird applesauce brownie, you will relapse to having the real brownie, and go on another sugar roller coaster.

Let's be completely on board with the food plan, and not leave a little part of us not all in, because those are the parts that scream the loudest when we are stuck at the airport and we see Starbucks selling brownies the size of a phone book. It is better to leave all the old tastes behind. Think of it as a cleaner breakup; we are returning all of their stuff, defriending them on social media, and deleting them from our phone. Do not leave any door open to get back together with sugar. You deserve better.

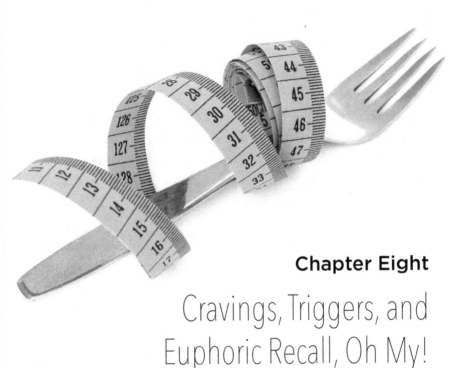

Chapter Eight

Cravings, Triggers, and Euphoric Recall, Oh My!

MUCH LIKE THE LIONS, tigers, and bears to be afraid of in *The Wizard of Oz*, we need to be concerned with avoiding cravings, triggers, and euphoric recall. Let's tackle them one by one.

Cravings

These are rather controversial. Some natural types will tell you that a craving for something sweet means you are low in a particular vitamin. Other nutrition folks will say if you have a craving for something sweet, try to appease it with beets or carrots. You know, give it a little of what you really want to see if that soothes the savage Sugar Beast. I say none of these approaches work.

If you are experiencing a desire for a Twinkie, it does not mean you are low in a particular nutrient as Twinkies are devoid of all nutrients and vitamins. If you just got stuck in traffic and thought of Twinkies the entire time, it is not a sign you need to have a little bit of one, or to try and do the faux approach, and have a bowl of carrots and pretend it is a Twinkie. When you walk into a gas station running late and need to get a tank of gas, and see Twinkies and think that would be a great idea, again it is not a craving – it is a bad habit. When you take your three-year-old daughter to the library and think of Twinkies on the drive home, it does not necessarily mean you are low in magnesium or calcium. These are all examples of habits. If you were one of my own clients, we would talk in depth about why Twinkies meant so much to you – what it is about them. Usually it is something like your mom used to give them to you on Fridays after the library when you would walk home together holding hands, and you have warm, fuzzy memories when you think about Twinkies. So when you are stressed, your mind goes to the familiar space of Twinkies – where the acceptance and the hugs live. A bunch of chemicals and fake ingredients live there as well. These ideas going through your mind are not directives from a higher power or a mandatory sign from your body that you must "listen" to. It is a habit we must move past, and when you are having a bad day and need a boost, let's reminisce about the loving walk home with Mom, instead of taking a deep Hostess dive. You will never regret reminiscing or journaling about Mom, you will regret getting back on the sugar merry-go-round.

Triggers

Trigger is not just the name of the Lone Ranger's horse, but can in fact be a huge roadblock in our final breakup with sugar. The exact definition: A trigger is any form of stimuli that initiates the desire to engage in addictive behavior. During the course of a recovery program, triggers may prompt an individual to slip up and engage in a behavior that they otherwise are trying to avoid.

Let me tell you a story of when I really screwed up and what I learned. I was 21 days off of sugar and I had gotten into an argument with my husband over an event that he swore he'd told me about and I'd said I did not want to go. He never told me and I only knew about it when I smelled cologne and then saw him coming down the stairs in a suit one Saturday night when we did not have a babysitter. Earlier in the day, my daughter said she wanted me to help her make cupcakes. He left for the event, and I helped her make the cupcakes. Buttercream frosting is a problem for me when I am in a good mood, even if I wasn't newly off of sugar. Baking was always a sugar party for me. I loved cookie dough and batter in general. I believe salmonella is a cruel rumor started by the Fun Police. So, I had some frosting. I figured I was good since I "only" had a few tablespoons. However, I was still mad at myself, and I spent the next three days feeling like absolute crap, and the sugar cravings came back with a vengeance. Oh and my husband was still wrong. I had absolutely no business going anywhere near baking, even if I wasn't in an agitated state of mind: it was too soon after my sugar breakup since that was where I often got into trouble.

We all have different triggers. Mine are probably not the same as yours. Figure out what yours are and figure out practical solutions to work around them. This means I do not bake anymore, or eat any food that is not mine, as I used to always eat my kids' leftover food, which was an issue with my inability to lose weight, and, let's be honest here, flat-out gross.

Euphoric Recall

Our brain doesn't know that sugar is socially acceptable and cocaine could land you in prison or at least rehab. Remember how sugar is eight times more addictive than cocaine? Euphoric recall is an issue no matter what the substance. It directly affects an area of the brain called the pleasure or reward center. This is the same part of the brain that manages a variety of important psychological functions such as the following: emotional response, anxiety management, reinforcing behaviors (forming habits), the ability to resist impulses, the formation and recollection of memories. Remember the frosting from a few paragraphs ago? I remember the buttercream frosting tasted amazing, not the normal sort of frosting taste. Euphoric recall loaded the flavor with extra pleasure. It did not last long because my logical brain caught up to my reward center and I remembered how much I did not want this in my life. I thought about how miserable I was before, and I immediately started to regret what I had done. I envisioned Times Square on New Year's Eve as my reward center. Ryan Seacrest and the giant ball were there. I was shouting "We broke up," in the middle of the gigantic crowd and no one was listening because everyone else was having a giant pleasure party.

This is why it is so important to avoid euphoric recall from having "just a bite" or falling for the moderation myth. Look back on all the false starts you had, and I bet you can think back to what particular food item did it. I remember going to Disney World with my daughter in late October one year and I was being so "good" on Weight Watchers. I had started again in early September and I was the living and breathing example of perfection when it came to discipline. That was, until we went to the water park and there was a layered sundae with bacon. I remember even calling my husband at work to tell him about it since he loves bacon. My daughter offered me a bite and I said "OK" to the ice cream, even though I knew better, even though I had been "good" for weeks. I basically took a ten-pound bite with that sundae. I don't remember being on track again until after the holidays, as I kept kicking the can down the road.

It Is 5 O'clock Somewhere

I do not care about alcohol, I never consume it unless the other person is, I have a hard time finishing a drink, and even if I have it in my house, it would never occur to me to open it up. Even if I got a speeding ticket or found out my ex-boyfriend married a supermodel, I wouldn't go to the wine I had in my house.

However, if I had a giant serving of sugar on Saturday, I am 99 percent sure I would be a flipping mess on Tuesday. This is because Sunday would have been worse than Saturday night, Sunday would have morphed into Monday, and by Tuesday I would be bloated, not able to think, have not just the chemical problems going on in my head with sugar, but all of my self-hatred, denial, why again, dieting-will-fix-it thought … and odds are, on Tuesday I would be a disaster.

Wine and champagne have high sugar contents, and if we eliminate all other types of sugar, do not think you can still have alcohol. However, many women would have a food day like I used to but finish with wine. Wine, simply put, is sugar. Remember, sugar creates cravings for more sugar. Let's take the alcohol dependency possibility out of the equation for a minute and talk purely about sugar issues. Ending the day with a ton of sugar will only feed the sugar-demanding villi in your stomach, the sugar chemicals in your brain, and the sugar habit in your overall being.

Other Obstacles and My Strategies

Now, there are many real life obstacles my clients and I have run into and I want to share the strategies with you.

- I always have the minibar cleared out when I go to a hotel. I do not need the Toblerone calling my name at two in the morning.
- I try to eat pretty much the same, every day, all year. Not so I pass out from boredom, but to stop the association of food with celebrations.

- I stick to a sleep routine the best I can. I do not eat too close to bedtime, which is easier to do when you know when you are going to sleep.
- I have a kit I travel with. It always has packaged albacore tuna, soy nuts, RX bars, and nuts. I do not want to have to eat this for days, but I have been in some strange places where I found only low quality or potentially triggering offerings.
- To the well-meaning food pusher, just say, "No, thanks," or "I am good." Do not get into a discussion with her or him about the poison that is sugar or why you can't just have one.
- Everyone is ordering dessert or coffee. Get hot water and lemon or tea.
- You are stuck in an airport and have no idea what you can eat. Ninety-nine percent of the time you can always find a chicken breast or beef patty. Add grilled onions and avocado. Hold the bread and have a couple of sweet potato fries. Have a big salad with full-leaded dressing.
- You are on a flight and the only thing they are offering is packaged bags of chemicals and sugar. Say no thanks. This is between meals and you can survive. If it was a mealtime, you could have planned ahead and brought back-ups.
- Someone hands you cake at a kid's birthday party. They insist you have some, you pass it to the next husband you see when they walk by. It never fails.
- There is a cookie swap party you are invited to. I would cruise by a bakery on the way to the party as baking isn't conducive to my breakup with sugar.
- Your kid made you something special. Say you will eat it later or say thank you and make your spouse eat it or the dog. Either one is fine.

- When in doubt, know that no one can make you eat anything you do not want to.
- My favorite go-tos that have gotten me out of many situations are "I just brushed my teeth," or "I just ate." No one reasonable can argue with those.

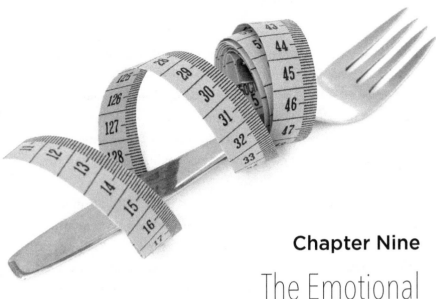

Chapter Nine

The Emotional Elephant in the Room

Did I Hit a Nerve?

When I was studying to become a food addiction counselor, I put something on social media about the process. It wasn't overly obnoxious, it was something like #foodaddictionexists after a string of five or six other hashtags.

A friend of mine, Monica, who owns a small exercise studio in my community took me aside the next chance she got to tell me how I can't post anything like that again or else she wouldn't recommend me to any of her clients. Not only was I in total shock, I immediately became intrigued as to why I hit such a nerve with Monica. Thankfully, I said I appreciated her feedback. I told her what I had been studying and all the issues with food I have personally experienced, and what twelve-step food groups I had attended to gain additional insight.

A few days later, Monica texted me asking when she could go to the twelve-step meeting and then blew up my phone with questions as to what she could eat and what was going on with her own eating habits. She is the only person in my world who has ever mentioned being a food addiction counselor as a negative.

I do not always enter a client meeting or a professional situation with food addiction in neon flashing lights, because I know it can put people off. I am also a holistic health coach, which is a little more tolerable for the average person. I have a great deal of theoretical knowledge and real life experience in food addiction and its evil twin sister, emotional eating.

Wrestling with Shame

There is one word that brings terror to a mother like nothing else and I know this because I lived through it and I survived. It is a four-letter word, and the problem is it isn't discussed enough and if people would just talk about it, so much of the problem would be contained and the shame would stop. What is this I am referring to? LICE.

My kids had just changed schools and earlier in the summer, my daughter was complaining her head itched, and we were at the beach, and I looked at it and it was sand (or so I thought). She had just finished eight weeks of day camp and at the time, her hair was to the middle of her back. Fast forward a few weeks and the new school does lice checks. Both of our kids had it so bad, they were immediately quarantined in the nurse's office at the new school. My husband was called from work to come and get the kids. We all know how bad it is when your husband leaves the office!

I went through my phone and figured out what playdates and birthday parties the kids had attended recently. I immediately called all the new friends my kids had made and said "Hey! Guess what? Remember me, Erin Wathen? Funny thing, my kid probably gave you lice. I am so sorry."

My daughter had generations in her hair. Remember the "sand" I saw? It is too gross for words, and as I write this I feel psychosomatic itching happening up and down my head. A long and expensive story later, we all had a few, our daughter won gold medal hands down, our entire house had to be bug bombed, and I totally went nuts getting everything cleaned. I became absolutely obsessive with washing backpacks, coats, not going to movie theaters, and spraying the kids' stuff with lice spray.

Since the lice lady who came over to help me and I became great friends in her marathon session with our family, she and I got talking about why lice is such a huge problem in the NYC suburbs. A few reasons: First, people travel from all over the world, so certain strains are brought from all over the world; secondly, places such as camps are very densely populated so the bugs can easily spread; and lastly, secrecy and shame. Shame I said? What? Keep in mind it was around 4 a.m. and I had been up since 6 a.m. and I was a nervous wreck. She explained to me that a large part of the problem is that when a child has lice, the parents are embarrassed, and they don't tell the other families. The other kids do not get checked when it might not have been very bad, and by the time it gets noticed, the entire other family has it. This happens all the time, she said.

This got me thinking about what Brené Brown says about shame, "Shame needs three things to grow exponentially in our lives: secrecy, silence, and judgment." Now, let's face it, lice happens. Even to nice people, even to us!

So, if everyone I knew that had a kid with lice would have simply told the school, the soccer team, and the friends, it would stop spreading. The shame wouldn't have a fighting chance.

Emotional Eating

Emotional eating also has a strong stink of shame associated with it. Everyone does it, but few will admit it. Of course, I will, but I am an open book. Hell, you are reading my open book!

We have all emotionally eaten. If you have ever had a piece of cake at a party, or stuffing on Thanksgiving, or candy corn on Halloween, you have eaten to celebrate an occasion, which is contradictory to consuming food to fuel your body. So, let's just destigmatize emotional eating right off the start. We have all done it to some degree, and there are many reasons why we eat in addition to hunger. It could be because everyone else at the table is eating chips at the Mexican restaurant.

I recently co-taught a workshop where I was the lead on the emotional eating section, and it made the group of women very nervous to even discuss the idea of emotional eating. I posted on the secret Facebook page and while I could tell everyone had read it, no one responded. Nevertheless, every group meeting would start with a talk about a recent obstacle in their weight loss journey, and the reason was always due to a personal relationship. Their marriage, a high maintenance sister-in-law, or a falling out with a long-time girlfriend…. These are all personal issues which had a direct correlation to their weight, and showed the connection between food and emotions.

The only problem food ever solves is hunger, so to use food to solve any other type of problem is a mistake because:

a. The original problem or issue isn't addressed.
b. Now you have the food to metabolize and 99 percent of the time we do not reach for broccoli when we are bored, restless, sad, or obsessing over something that happened at work. So now we have the emotions we haven't addressed, and the crappy food (which is almost always some sort of toxin) we are throwing at our body to try to handle it.

We aren't giving ourselves any nutrients nor the TLC we need to deal
with the emotions so the blows keep on coming.

How do I tell emotional hunger from physical hunger in myself?

1. Emotional hunger comes on super strong. Let's use this example: I spoke to my Mom and now I want ice cream. I need ice cream now. I need it so badly, I am eating it while on the phone with her. If someone comes in the room, I am embarrassed and I act as though I am not eating the ice cream. I do not want an apple or a kale salad. Only ice cream would satisfy me.

2. When I have the ice cream, I feel guilty about it. I am ashamed of my choice.

3. I do not even realize I have eaten the whole container until it is done. I tell myself it doesn't really matter since I worked out today, but this clearly matters. I am going through a whole mental game trying to make it OK that I ate this. Would I be doing this over chicken? Or ice cream I ate with other humans rather than in the dark? (I'm still not assigning any bandwidth to the issue with Mom, since I have a new problem.)

4. After I have acknowledged that I consumed the ice cream, my mind goes to how I can make up for the ice cream. (Still nothing about Mom.)

5. For the next day or two, I am so busy being consumed with self-loathing and over-exercising and under-eating, I do not address the emotions that were stirred up during the phone call with Mom. Look, I have a problem I am a little more OK with addressing: the ramifications of the ice cream. I am not sleeping well as my body is trying to handle all the sugar, the chemicals in the protein Halo Top thing, and all the stress I am putting on my body by doing doubles at the gym. (Still no time to think about my Mom, too busy weighing my carrots.)

How many times have you done this? I have at least 1,000 times. I used to think ice cream was the problem, if only I could find a way to live in a world without ice cream then everything would be fine. Now, I realize ice cream was only a symptom and if I try and *not* feel my feelings, it will only lead to bigger problems down the line.

Do you remember the song "Going on a Bear Hunt" from childhood? It is the kind of thing you would have sung at camp or in primary school. The narrators are going to look for bears and things keep getting in their way. They encounter things like bridges, mud, fences, snowstorms, and finally they find the bear cave. The premise is you can't go around the obstacle, under the obstacle, or over the obstacle – you have to go through the obstacle. This is how we must face our feelings. I should have never gone to the ice cream after the conversation with my mother. I was creating a new problem to solve, one I was more comfortable with solving than the one I needed to address, the issues with my mom. I could have gotten out my journal, gone and talked to my husband, called my brother to vent, caught up with my DVR, gone for a workout… there were about 1,000 things I could have done other than create a new problem and distract myself with food.

To be fair, how familiar were these patterns in my brain? How strong was this bad habit? This is what I had conditioned myself to do. It had worked for decades, as much as a bad habit can work. It took a while to fully stop this pattern, and I had to be kind to myself during the process. Expecting immediate results wasn't realistic or kind to myself.

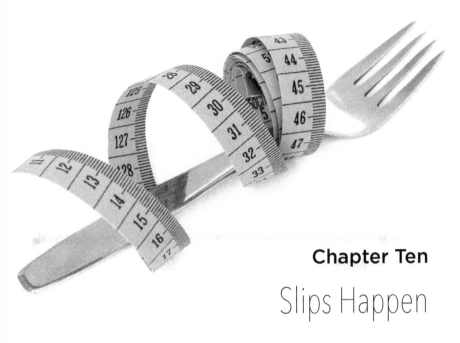

Chapter Ten

Slips Happen

DESPITE YOUR BEST INTENTIONS, there might be a time when you eat the churro or the frosting or the cake at the wedding. Now, what do you do?

Let's say you have been doing the *Break Up with Sugar* method for the last 75 days, and you had really hit your groove. Nevertheless, you were feeling really anxious about a big presentation at work that was coming up, your friend who quit sugar years ago had to cancel at the last minute to meet up due to a sick kid, and instead of walking directly into the movie theater, you glance over to the concession stand, there isn't a line, and you see a familiar face behind the register. You go over to say hi to your neighbor Rachel, the teenage girl employed at the snack bar – she is such a nice kid after all. The next thing you know you got your usual, well your old usual. Half way through the giant box of Milk Duds, after you had already demolished the Junior Mints in record time, your peace-loving thoughts catch up to your reward mind and put the brakes on the whole thing. It is as if you wake up from the sugar daze and are immediately thrown by what just happened and how quickly you fell into your old ways. Your thoughts are all over the place, you might be thinking things such as "Did the last 75 days mean nothing?" "How come other people can ditch sugar and you can't?" or "Would it really be so bad to just finish the stinking Milk Duds, the day is already ruined?"

The last 75 days show you are capable of showing great discipline, ability, and focus. To throw them away and guzzle the Milk Duds would be the equivalent of slashing three good tires because one is flat. It is illogical, but when we are upset, our hijacked brains can go to some dark places.

Let's reframe the slip as a teaching tool, and see what we could have done differently. Knowing we were anxious about the presentation at work, having our friend cancel at the last minute is enough of a warning for us to be extra vigilant in our resolve to stay broken up with sugar. We started doing the slow dance of lying to ourselves when we glanced at the concession stand at all. Would this have happened if our friend had met us and her kid had not been sick? Probably not. As soon as you walked toward the concession stand, let's be honest, you knew where things were headed. This is like calling the ex at 2 a.m. to say you miss them, we all know what that call is – a booty call. Saying hello to the girl behind the counter was nice, but it wasn't necessary, you could have waved. It is crucial that we own our slips. If we start blaming our friend's kid for being sick and the friend for not showing up, Rachel the teenage girl for being friendly, or the people who invented Junior Mints, there will be no growth from this slip and the lesson will be lost in a sea of finger pointing, shame, and blaming.

On the flip side, if we go into a shame pit, it is equally damaging. A friend of mine was newly off of sugar for a few months, had a rotten day, ate a carton of Ben and Jerry's, and became hysterical due to being so sick of fighting her sugar issues. Thankfully, she called a sugar-free friend and was able to quit sugar for good and has maintained it for 15 years.

Having a slip happens to some people, however they do not have to keep happening if you are open to learning from them. Be aware of any strange feelings and cravings you have for the next three days or so as your body tries to handle the sugar it was once so fond of. Also, you could be fighting the urge go back to sugar more than usual. You will survive, but you will not be any smarter if you are not too willing to learn the lesson of what you could have done.

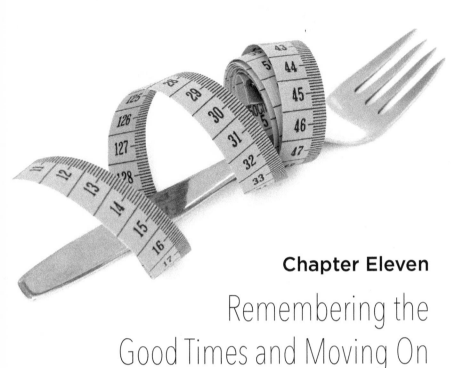

Chapter Eleven

Remembering the Good Times and Moving On

NOW AFTER A BAD BREAKUP, we all tend to dwell on how awful the other person was. Then there comes a time where we get sentimental remembering all the "good" times. I remember re-reading all my high school boyfriend's love letters after he dumped me for being needy. Not sure why I decided to pour salt in my wound, but it seems to be one of the steps we all go through.

As much as it pains me to write this, sugar did serve a purpose. There were times when sugar did help, for example with my Mom and the feelings I did not want to feel. So let's rewind that same scenario and imagine I did not have the ice cream. How would I have felt? I would have had to sit with those crappy feelings and that stinks. It is much easier, or so it seemed, to stuff those awful ideas in a sea of Chubby

Hubby than to acknowledge the anger, disappointment, or frustration I had at the time.

A Promise Kept

When you started this journey with me, I promised you a few things. Specifically these:

- You would learn why diets are so hard to stick to. We have gone over why they are so difficult: the stinking white stuff we see and the lurking white stuff just waiting to hijack our brains and our good intentions. It is not a matter of being good people, which I am, you know, most of the time – unless some kid wrongs my kid but other than that you are in the clear – but brain chemistry. Moderation does not work with the white stuff; our friends the rats showed us that.

- What is preventing us from sticking to our diets. Well, we know it was not a lack of knowledge as to how many calories are in a four-ounce skinless boneless chicken breast (184). It was not the desire, since we had been trying since, you know, a week before forever. It was the sugar, the flour, and the artificial sweeteners that were undermining our efforts, time and time again.

- How I learned to stick to my diet by not being on a diet. Food plans are life. They are not good or bad, they just are. I am neither starving myself nor eating in the dark. I am eating three good-sized meals a day and I do not have an emotional reaction or physical reaction to my food, other than being fueled for my life.

- Living the rest of your life not on a diet, yet maintaining your weight loss. My scale has read the same, give or take within two pounds for two years. The two pounds depends on the time of the month, or if I have been drinking enough water. Given how

I could lose or gain seven pounds in a week in the old days, this is a modern-day miracle to me. This will happen to you, once you break up with all the sugars.

- We will figure out a specialized food plan for the rest of your life. You might not eat exactly how I eat, you might love eggs, for example. However, the concepts are the same. No white stuff. Keep supplies in your car or bag just in case. Ask questions to the waiter, do not be afraid to stand up for what you know is best for yourself.

- You will learn how to combat any food obstacle. Go to the list at the end of Chapter Seven for any and all food obstacles. Take a picture of the list with your phone and use it at a party. When in doubt, nicely tell the sugar pusher "no, thanks." Resist the urge to ask them, "What the hell is your problem?" No good will come of that, other than you might feel better for three seconds, and then regret it.

- You will learn to ditch the diet mentality for good. You have. No more diets to stick to as there will be no more diets. No more "I-am-seeing-my-best-friend-next-week-and-need-to-drop-ten-pounds-fast diet," or the "Spring-break-is-coming-up-and-I-forgot-I cannot-fit-into-any-of-my-shorts diet," or "The-polar-vortex-made-me-and-bread-BFFs-for-life diet." You get the idea. We are done with diets, the white stuff, having three pairs of the same style of pants in our closet, the sugar drama, the food drama, the acne, the low grade depression, the mood swings, the numerous health risks, and feeling bad about ourselves. We are *done*.

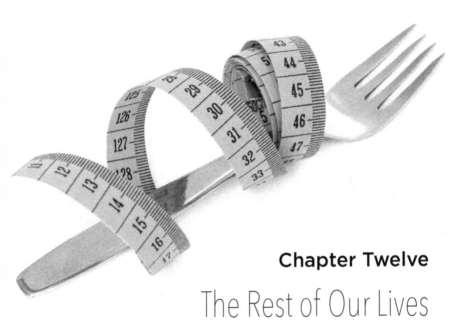

Chapter Twelve

The Rest of Our Lives

THEY CALL THE FIRST couple of weeks of being sugar-free "living on a pink cloud." Everything seems so much better, life is easier, and full of unicorns and rainbows. However, right around day 21, the clouds come in and the unicorns move on to someone else's yard. You might have this false sense of "I've got this." You have a fabulous idea that you can be one of those magical creatures, much like a unicorn, who can have some sugar. Well, you can't. I write this with all the love in the world, but you need to remember your #1 Why. If you start thinking you have not had 1000 failed attempts at sticking to your diet, open up envelope Why #2 if you still believe you can have just a bite. Go all the way to #5 if you have any more ideas of having a faux brownie. Then go back up and do it again.

Sugar makes us want more sugar, plain and simple. It makes us bloated, moody, and it hijacks our brain into thinking more sugar will make it all better. Sugar pretends it is our friend, when it is in fact our worst enemy. Sugar has done more to damage the health of Americans than even cigarettes. The obesity rates in America track identically to the increased consumption of processed foods and drinks whose first ingredient is sugar.

After decades of falling for this lie, I realized sugar did not make things better; in fact, it always made them worse, but for a few minutes it gave me false hope. When the feel-good parts of my brain were lighting up like a Christmas tree, it was amazing – however, when the lights left, I had to go back to the crappy situation I was trying to hide from. Now what sort of a friend does that? A bad friend, the sort of friend you eventually realize is toxic and you break up with. Much like I had to do with sugar.

Why was this final time different? Because I didn't do it for anyone but myself. I didn't do it for a bikini or to have a six-pack by spring break. I did it so I could start living in peace. My Why had to be different. It couldn't be short-term and it had to be internal. Once I connected with my Why, I could become a better mother, wife, friend, and human being, However, my family really didn't care or notice if I weighed twelve pounds less or not. They did notice if I was extra special moody because I was full of self-loathing, or if I was testy at drop off because I needed to get to the spin class to get rid of whatever I had done to myself the night before when no one was looking.

I realized I didn't crave sugar once I started eating high fat/low carb. I had to experiment, but the 40/40/20 macro breakdown works best to eliminate sugar for me and my clients. Now, there is a period of social adjustment to a life of high fat/low carb – however, would you rather be in sugar hell and have the churro or live in peace? These are the questions I ask myself. I always pick peace; I pick peace because it lasts much longer than the short-term satisfaction of the churro. The churro will be eaten in five minutes or so, but the consequences would last for at least three days – if not weeks, depending on whether it triggered me or not. Let's assume it did in fact trigger me – would it be worth it then? Remember, sugar is a progressive situation so it will take more and more of it to have the same level of satisfaction. It wouldn't be that long before I was drowning in a sea of white stuff in my pantry at 11 p.m. while my family was asleep. The candy bags would reappear in the center console of my car as would the cavities I kept getting and my GI issues I never liked to talk about. I pick peace each and every time. I have had a lifetime of churros and I know what they taste like.

The physical adjustment to high fat/low carb takes a while as well. The first couple of days, you most likely would experience some headaches, lethargy, emotional distress, anger, and even nausea; all can be symptoms of withdrawal from sugar. Drink lots of water and get more sleep than usual; do not put yourself in any especially tempting situations. Now is not the time to decorate cookies or to test every type of shortbread on your trip to Scotland. Be especially kind to yourself – I cannot emphasize that enough. You will have years of habits of physically walking to the concessions at the movies, or of always getting a giant Rainbow Snow Cone at the local festival each August. How about you use this as an opportunity to find new traditions that do not involve food? I always tell my clients to look at this as a good time for new traditions. I have to be careful when I say this, as if they are early in detox, or they are likely to not hear me and roll their eyes.

The emotional adjustment is a tough one – I am not going to sugarcoat it (sorry). We went to food because it was fun, and someone we loved gave it to us, the commercials on TV had smiling kids with popsicles, and it isn't like the ice cream man sold green beans. Sugar meant fun. Sugar meant celebration. Sugar meant love. However, sugar came to mean a hijacked brain and mood swings. Sugar meant needing more and more. Sugar meant being in a constant state of shame if someone found out what I really ate. Sugar was my best friend and my worst enemy. We had become toxic and had to break up. Sugar didn't go without a fight. Sugar is a stage five clinger. However, peace is worth it. Obsessing about what you are going to do in six months at Derek and Jane's wedding during the cake cutting is not going to help you today. All you can be concerned with is what you are going to eat today and maybe tomorrow through your meal planning. You had an emotional relationship with sugar and it was there for you when you didn't want to deal with the bad grade you got on the midterm in Anthropology, or when you and your boyfriend got into a big fight over politics, and sometimes you just needed it because you had a headache, or because it could be fun.

It is understandable and appropriate to grieve the loss of something or someone you believed to be your friend. So if you need to mourn losing sugar, give yourself space to do so. Have a good cry, go out on a run, complain to a trusted friend, or go buy a pair of shoes in memoriam. Honor your feelings, but don't let this grief go on for more than a day or two. I let my clients direct it all to me because I get it, and many times the other people in our lives don't. And even if the people in our lives support us whole-heartedly, we still might not feel comfortable breaking down over the churros we will never get to have.

It might help to remind yourself that in what you perceive as loss, there is so much more to gain. In giving up sugar, you will get your life, your mind, and your health back. See it as a visual: everything you want from your life on one side, and a sticky pile of empty calories and dangerously addictive junk food on the other. When you can truly see it like this, it no longer feels like a sacrifice. You get *you* back. And that is worth more than all the churros in the world.

Appendix

Pantry staples

OILS AND FATS

Coconut oil: I use coconut oil for my primary cooking oil. It's a saturated fat that's solid at room temperature, making it incredibly stable when heat is applied. It won't break down and oxidize like monounsaturated fats such as olive oil. Always choose virgin, unrefined coconut oil.

Extra virgin olive oil: Be aware that many olive oils have been cut with soy and vegetables oils, so make sure what you're buying is true olive oil. Olive oil should be used for low and medium temp cooking. I also like the flavored olive oils infused with garlic, basil, or lemon.

Ghee: I always have Ghee on hand, I am cool with Trader Joe's and it will last a long time

MCT: (Medium Chain Triglycerides) oil is basically coconut oil on steroids. Bulletproof's Brain Octane Oil is 100-percent sourced from coconuts, so it's a very clean energy source and supports a healthy brain and metabolism.

NON PERISHABLES

What I currently have in my pantry-

Superfood toppings: unsweetened coconut, chia seeds, hemp seeds, pumpkin seeds, sunflower seeds: For puddings, salads, and garnishes.

Hemp Hearts: These are my new favorite thing. I have been using them on an avocado and them I put the whole thing in a broiler for breakfast. Google "what to do with hemp hearts" and see about 10 other cool ways to use them.

Nut Butters: I have at least 8 different types in my pantry, I counted. Try to stay away from peanut butter, they tend to have a bunch of junk in them, and they aren't as nutritious as tree nuts. My favorites are Cashew Butter and Macadamia. I love nut butter with fruit, or a smoothie or on a waffle or because it a great way to get fat/protein on the go.

Almonds, Pine Nuts, Cashews and Macadamia Nuts; be sure to store in glass jars

Soya Flour: I will make waffles from these or when I make a baked good. THe flour has protein, so it doesn't hit my blood stream in the same way flour does. However, I am very reluctant to use it very often. Other options include **whole spelt, almond flour and coconut flour.**

Cacao powder: for Freezer fudge and baking

Quinoa: A great grain alternative and it has protein

Black Bean Pasta: Sometimes, I want pasta, but I don't want flour. I will have this instead

Trader Joe's Coconut Granola: be careful, very calorically dense.

Dried Fruit: without any added sugars or oils. I like to keep dried raisins, currants, blueberries and dates on hand. Be careful with these as they are very calorically dense.

Fresh beans such as lentils, split peas, chick peas, kidney beans, and black beans: Can be used in soups, added to salads, made into fresh hummus, and used as a great source of protein on Meatless Mondays.

Tomatoes and Tomato paste in glass jars; Spaghetti sauce or chili

Coconut, Rice or Hemp Milk in tetra paks; For when you don't want to drink milk, and not as fussy with the expiration dates

Salad Dressings: A selection of vinegars for making your own dressing. My favorites include apple cider vinegar, rice vinegar, red wine vinegar, white wine vinegar, good quality balsamic and champagne vinegar mixed with unrefined olive oil.

Popcorn; Non GMO for Movie night

SWEETENERS

I do not use these on a regular basis, but I have a family and I know I need to upgrade meaning not use regular sugar when I bake: Less-offensive, unrefined sweeteners such as **brown-rice syrup, pure maple syrup, and coconut palm sugar.**

SPICES

A fresh stock of dried herbs and spices, preferably in glass jars. Some that I like to keep on hand include **cumin, oregano, coriander, chili powder, paprika, smoked paprika, garlic powder, onion powder, turmeric** and **cayenne**. For baking I always have cinnamon, ginger, nutmeg and cloves. Save some of the less common spices for when you need it for a specific recipe, that way they won't be hanging around your pantry for too long!

SALT

Always use **unrefined sea salt**. I get mine from Costco. Celtic sea salt is great for adrenal support.

TEA

I am a huge tea drinker. I always have green tea, matcha, Yogi bedtime tea and **AVEDA tea.**

My Refrigerator

Remember the MTV show Cribs where celebrities would show their homes and it always included a tour of the fridge? I still buy organic yogurt in a tube some added sugar in it for my 8 year old son. My husband's left over Duck Dumplings from the other night are in the back corner and he eats takeout less often than he used to. My 12 year old daughter still loves the funky little red waxy cheeses, so they stay. Our Hungarian Viszla has frozen organic treats I make her, and they look like meat whiz popsicles. If it was just my fridge, it would be different. Let's just say our family fridge isn't Cribs but my mini fridge in my office is a beautiful sight.

Moving on from my family and back to the essentials…

Kerrygold butter I worked for this company in my 20s before anyone had ever bought of making Bulletproof coffee. The best butter as far as I am concerned. It takes a while to get accustomed to the sizing.

Organic Milk, cream, yogurt and sour cream I try and use organic if available but I do not have a brand I look for specifically. I do not get skim ever.

Udi's bread I do not use it often, but I keep in the freezer.

Eggs- at least a dozen.

Poland Spring Seltzer I drink a ton of sparkling water in general. I will get the flavored ones if I can not find Poland Spring, but only the ones without anything funky in them. Stay away from the natural flavors added, you do not want those.

Fish- I buy as needed.

Organic beef and chicken- the beef I get a monthly delivery for and chicken from grocery store. Anything I will not use that day, I keep in the freezer.

Sauces and Condiments

Hot sauce all kinds, make sure sugar is not listed on the top 6 of the ingredients, or at all.

Capers I just love them, **Wasabi mayonaise**, sugar free Ketchup and reduced sodium **soy sauce.**

Vegetables

I am a big advocate for all things seasonal. Just because they sell cantaloupe in January in Connecticut does not mean I buy it. I always keep onions, carrots and celery in the fridge. Spinach, cucumbers, lemons and limes always make an appearance. I make a lot of salads in the summer, and soups in the winter. I do not have a longer list of vegetables I always keep because of my commitment to seasonal eating.

Freezer

Frozen Blueberries, mangoes and peaches- never hurts for a last minute smoothie or to add to yogurt.

Pre-portioned frozen onions, and basil- Trader Joe's carries a great brand. So handy for throwing in a soup or a marinara.

Sample Meal Plan

To keep it simple remember the basic 4:
1. Meal Planning
2. We eat from the perimeter of the grocery store:
    1. Fruits
    2. Vegetables
    3. Meats, Fish, Eggs and Vegetable Proteins
    4. Dairy (If you can tolerate it)*
3. Three meals a day
4. Every time you eat, we check these 4 boxes
    1. Protein
    2. Fat
    3. Low Glycemic Carbohydrate
    4. Fiber

*Butter should be used to cook with, along with Oil/Ghee

A few things to remember:
1. The reasoning behind low glycemic fruit in the morning is to keep our blood sugar even throughout the day.
2. I drink water, tea or seltzer all day. I can't handle black coffee. If you can, you are my hero. I can't stomach it. So, have at it.

3. Lunch *should* be the largest meal of your day. I TRY, which doesn't always happen especially when life gets lifey. To have fish or chicken at night vs. beef, as I find it to be heavier.
4. After dinner, you are done. The KITCHEN IS CLOSED
5. The portion sizes are mine. If you are a 100 lb. woman who is pretty sedentary, you are not going to need to eat as much as a 225 lb. man who is training for a ToughMudder. Experiment with what feels right for you.
6. I recommend weighing and measuring for a week or two, no matter what your goals are.
7. Unlimited Vegetables include everything in the produce section. Except for Potatoes, Corn, and Carrots. I would have those every so often, but in a small amount and at lunch, and also not for the first couple of weeks.
1. All of my meals include Fat. The vegetables are sautéed in coconut oil, the salad dressing is fully leaded and I use real butter with artichokes. I don't use Pam or diet anything.
2. I do not get too specific with what exactly you should eat, as I do not know what you like
   10. Glycemic Index Link
   https://www.health.harvard.edu/diseases-and-conditions/glycemic-index-and-glycemic-load-for-100-foods

Food Plan

Breakfast
Protein 4-6 oz
Fruit 8oz
Low glycemic carb
Fat

Lunch
Protein 6 oz
Vegetables UNLIMITED
Low glycemic carb
Fat

Dinner
Protein 6 oz
Vegetables UNLIMITED
Low glycemic carb

My Food Last Week

Breakfast
- Spinach and sausage, sautéed vegetables with cheese, grapefruit
- Soy waffle with berries, and almond butter

- Cherry Chicken Sausage, side of sautéed vegetables

Lunch

- Hamburger patty, grilled onions, crumbled blue cheese, a few sweet potato fries
- Caprese salad, chicken breast, side salad W/dressing
- Grilled swordfish, sautéed spinach with pine nuts, Zoodles

Dinner

- Filet mignon, grilled asparagus, spinach salad w/dressing
- Shredded beef, green salsa salsa, avocado, grilled vegetables
- Turkey breast, sautéed kale with pine nuts and a few raisins

Glycemic index

http://www.glycemicindex.com

The **glycemic index** or (**GI**) is a number associated with the carbohydrates in a particular type of food that indicates the effect of these carbohydrates on our blood sugar level. A value of 100 represents the standard, an equivalent amount of pure glucose.

The GI represents the rise in a person's blood sugar level two hours after consumption of the food. The glycemic effects of foods depends on a number of factors, such as the type of carbohydrate, physical entrapment of the carbohydrate molecules within the food, fat and protein content of the food and organic acids or their salts in the meal. The GI is useful for understanding how the body breaks down carbohydrates and takes into account only the available carbohydrate (total carbohydrate minus fiber) in a food. Glycemic index does not predict an individual's glycemic response to a food, but can be used as a tool to assess the insulin response burden of a food, averaged across a studied population. Individual responses vary greatly.

Further Reading

Food Junkies: The Truth About Food Addiction by Vera Tarman

Grain Brain: The Surprising Truth about Wheat, Carbs, and Sugar: Your Brain's Silent Killer by David Perlmutter and Kristin Robert

Wheat Belly: Lose the Wheat, Lose the Weight, and Find Your Path Back To Health by William Davis

Breaking Free From Emotional Eating by Geneen Roth

Acknowledgments

I am thankful for my husband for putting up with me when I was writing this. He always believed in me when I was having my moments of doubt, when I wanted to crawl back into bed and buy expensive shoes online. I still like to do that, but that is beside the point.

I am extremely grateful for my kids for tolerating me when I was living everything that went into this book. I look back and think of how distracted I was with the constant food noise in my brain and am glad that I was able to figure it out before they became teenagers and I needed to pay much better attention.

I wanted to give a shout out to my Mother who always told me I was a good writer, even when I was ten, had the world's worst handwriting, but had something to say. She gave me the confidence to start writing back in the days of a word processor, and was always willing to proofread my papers.

Words cannot express how much I need to acknowledge Dr. G. He would never admit it of course, which makes me appreciate him more.

I wanted to give a shout-out to my mentors in the Wellness world – Bethenny Frankel, Geneen Roth, and Jane Fonda – for always giving me inspiration.

A huge thank you to Olga, Terri and Marco. They make my life run smoothly.

I can not express the gratitude I have towards The Author Incubator and the legendary Angela Lauria. Her amazing reputation does not do her justice.

To the Morgan James Publishing team: Special thanks to David Hancock, CEO & Founder for believing in me and my message. To my Author Relations Manager, Gayle West, thanks for making the process seamless and easy. Many more thanks to everyone else, but especially Jim Howard, Bethany Marshall, and Nickcole Watkins.

The other day, my about-to-be-a-third-grader son was upset because he "did not know what he wanted to be when he grew up." I tried to take his existential crisis seriously, but I was thinking, "How long did it take me until I realized what I wanted to do?" About the same amount of time it took me to get my food together. The two are tied together in my mind. I could not have found my voice to write this book and to help others if I had not been through the countless diets, the trips up and down the scale, and the numerous Monday-morning diets. So, I am thankful to myself for never giving up. For after all of the craziness I put myself through, for believing there had to be a better way of living. I just had to find it.

About the Author

Erin grew up in California, went to college in Oregon and graduate school in Hawaii, and has been in the New York area for the last 15 years.

After working in a professional setting in Manhattan, Erin moved with her husband and children to the suburbs of New York. An avid exerciser, Erin started teaching group fitness while her children were young. Erin became a Holistic Health Coach through the Institute of Integrative Nutrition. During this

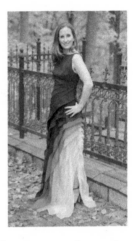

process became intrigued by food addiction, and was accepted into the INFACT program based out of Reykjavik, Iceland.

Erin spent the majority of her life wrestling with her sugar issues, and is happily now sugar free! She currently lives with her husband, two kids, the world's oldest cat and a hyperactive dog.

Website: www.ewwellnesssolutions.com

Email: erin@ewwellnesssolutions.com

-Why not ↓ carb dressings? - ↓ fat mary: Bumble+ Brown
- Yogurt dressing?

Thank You

I so much appreciate you taking the time to read Why Can't I Stick to My Diet? This is the end of your ugly breakup with sugar, but the beginning of your life free from diets, Monday-morning regrets, and having three sizes of the same pair of pants in your closet.

Visit ewwellnesssolutions.com so we can start a conversation and I can assist you with your own breakup with sugar. I am available to speak to groups.

In Good Health,

Erin

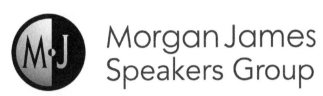

Morgan James
Speakers Group

We connect Morgan James published
authors with live and online events
and audiences who will benefit
from their expertise.

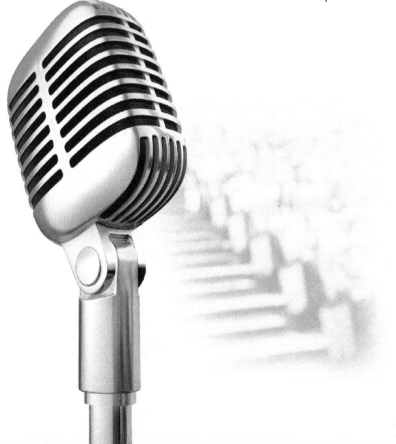

 Morgan James makes all of our titles available
through the Library for All Charity Organization.

www.LibraryForAll.org